Medical Analogy in Latin Satire

Also by Sari Kivistö

In Finnish:

LITERATURE IN CLASSICAL ANTIQUITY *(with H. K. Riikonen, Erja Salmenkivi and Raija Sarasti-Wilenius)*
CULTURE IN CLASSICAL ANTIQUITY *(with Mika Kajava, H. K. Riikonen, Erja Salmenkivi and Raija Sarasti-Wilenius)*
INTRODUCTION TO THE HISTORY AND THEORY OF SATIRE *(editor)*
ORNITHOLOGY AT THE ACADEMY OF TURKU *(with Esa Lehikoinen, Risto Lemmetyinen and Timo Vuorisalo)*

Medical Analogy in Latin Satire

Sari Kivistö
Ph.D., Docent

palgrave
macmillan

First published 2009 by
PALGRAVE MACMILLAN

Palgrave Macmillan in the UK is an imprint of Macmillan Publishers Limited, registered in England, company number 785998, of Houndmills, Basingstoke, Hampshire RG21 6XS.

Palgrave Macmillan in the US is a division of St Martin's Press LLC, 175 Fifth Avenue, New York, NY 10010.

Palgrave Macmillan is the global academic imprint of the above companies and has companies and representatives throughout the world.

Palgrave® and Macmillan® are registered trademarks in the United States, the United Kingdom, Europe and other countries.

ISBN: 978–0–230–22812–2 hardback

This book is printed on paper suitable for recycling and made from fully managed and sustained forest sources. Logging, pulping and manufacturing processes are expected to conform to the environmental regulations of the country of origin.

A catalogue record for this book is available from the British Library.

A catalog record for this book is available from the Library of Congress.

10 9 8 7 6 5 4 3 2 1
18 17 16 15 14 13 12 11 10 09

Printed and bound in Great Britain by
CPI Antony Rowe, Chippenham and Eastbourne

Si risus sanare potest, cur fletibus utar?
[If laughter can heal, why should I use tears?]

(Jacob Balde, *De eclipsi solari*, poem 44)

Contents

Acknowledgements ix

1 Introduction: Medicine for the Sick Soul 1
The analogy 4
Shared goals of satire and moral philosophy 7
The satirist as an expert healer 11
Internally sick: appetites as diseases 16
Hidden wounds and symptomatic colours in Roman satire 20
Changing traditions: from rotten insides to disease encomia 27

2 Medical Meta-language: Renaissance Commentaries and Poetics on the Healing Nature of Satire 32
Medicine as a metaphor for writing satire 32
The healing doctor and the sick doctor 37
Heinsius and Volpi on satirical catharsis 41
Satirical effects and emotions 47
Therapy as punishment 54

3 Painfully Happy: Satirical Disease Eulogies and the Good Life 62
Epideictic rhetoric and paradoxical praises of disease 63
Fever as a moral disease 67
Divine gout dwells in wealth and luxury 74
Enduring pain like a Stoic 80
The blessings of gout 86
Matthaeus Czanakius: in praise of the itch 94
On old age 100

4 Wonderfully Unaware: Sensory Disabilities, Contemplation and Consolation 103
Blindness and sin 103
Blindness and insight 106
Guther, Passerat and Puteanus on blindness 110
Marten Schoock on deafness 120
On the wonderful lethargy 127
The ambivalence of intoxication 132

5 Outlook and Virtue: Morally Symptomatic Physical Peculiarities **141**
Albert Wichgreve's praise of dwarfs 143
Intellectual outlook and thinness in Jacob Balde's poetry 149
Strange student diseases 158
The art of farting 167

6 Satire as Therapy **170**

Appendix: The Anthologies Used in This Study 175

Notes 179

Bibliography 194

Index 209

Acknowledgements

When I was very young I had an annoying habit of refusing to eat unless *Alice in Wonderland* was read aloud to me. One evening my father, tired from his long day in the paper factory, said, "We must teach that girl to read by herself". So I started to learn the ABC book and its obscure stories of D-D-a-Duck and other creatures. I remember how hard it was to understand any of it. Those days are long past; the present work was written while I was a Fellow at the Helsinki Collegium for Advanced Studies at the University of Helsinki. I am deeply grateful to those members of the Collegium's international advisory board who have (twice) deemed my research worthy of support. I thank the administration of the Collegium (Juha Sihvola, Maria Soukkio and others) for making the Collegium a pleasant place to stay, and I thank all the fellows whom I have briefly come to know during the past few years. I thank Anneli Aejmelaeus for teaching me Hebrew, Alaric Hall for a symposium on morality and health, Merja-Liisa Hinkkanen for leaving me her office in which to move with my bird Felix, Päivi Pahta for arranging a seminar with me on medical terms in transition, my former research assistant Timo Pankakoski for doing a good job with Easter eggs, and Heli Tissari for occasional theatre evenings and seminars. At the Department of Comparative Literature, I thank Hannu Riikonen for keeping me busy with other book projects and Päivi Mehtonen for reading several chapters of this manuscript in its final phase. Glenda Goss is to be thanked for her wonderful help with the English language. The librarians at the National Library of Finland, the Heidelberg University Library, the Herzog August Bibliothek in Wolfenbüttel and the Staatsbibliothek in Berlin have been very helpful. I thank the publishers Palgrave Macmillan for including this little book in their publication programme. Many thanks to the publisher's anonymous referee for detailed and thoughtful comments, which I have tried to follow; I am grateful that someone has cared enough to think about these issues with me. And to my close ones I am warmly grateful for allowing me to listen to the music of the spheres.

1
Introduction: Medicine for the Sick Soul

In the dedication to his praise of an ass, *Laus asini*, Dutch humanist Daniel Heinsius (1580–1655) censured social evils and the world's sick condition in medical terms. His dedication was addressed to Ewald Schrevel, a professor of medicine at Leiden, whose expert opinion of the current age Heinsius sought: "Touch it and feel its pulse, will you? I'll bet that you'll agree with Democritus, saying that 'this is no longer mere error, this is disease'." (1629b, p. 2.)[1] As signs of the morbid condition of the contemporary world, Heinsius mentioned inverted values. Contempt was shown towards the virtuous and the learned, and everything that was noble or worthy of eternal fame was treated with disgust. Geniuses and salutary authors of the ilk of Hippocrates, Galen, Aristotle, Plutarch and Cicero were abhorred and treated as if they were mere waste products. In Heinsius's view, in his day everybody was merely chasing the shadow of an ass.[2]

Heinsius's rhetoric of universal sickness and the wrong notions of the multitude reflected a conventional humanistic set of values in his insistence on knowing ancient authors and complaining about the present barbaric state of higher education. Pathological terms were frequently used in this connection by humanists to describe the decline of classical learning or the decay of the world in general (cf. Kühlmann 1982, pp. 67–112). But what is more important here is that Heinsius's medical rhetoric, using terms of universal pathology, also summarised the view that satirists have often held of a society and its inhabitants. In interpreting its evils in pathological terms, diagnosing vices as diseases and describing the ubiquity of madness, authors of satires have frequently applied medical imagery in their art of moral castigation. Significantly, Heinsius's list of neglected authorities also included ancient philosophers and medical authors, who will have an important role in illustrating the medical analogies in this study.

The medical analogy between vices and physical diseases is an important tool with which to analyse the nature and functioning of satire. Throughout history, satirists have employed images of bodily weakness and diseases as indices of the human condition. Human beings have been represented as ailing patients suffering from physical illnesses that were analogies for mental and moral defects needing improvement and medical care. The sources of illnesses were usually found in questionable living habits. Among the Roman satirists, Lucilius (c. 180–102 BC) had already declared that "We see him who is sick in mind showing the mark of it on his body" (26, frg. 678; trans. E. H. Warmington). Horace (65–8 BC) playfully argued – echoing the Stoics – that hardly anyone was deemed sane or healthy, since the world of satire was crowded with sick people (*Sermones* 2.3.32). Humanity's sick condition was specified as the reason for writing satires. Horace stated that vices were so common that anyone picked at random from a crowd was probably plagued with either avarice or some disease of ambition (*Sermones* 1.4.25–6). Even the impulse to write was considered a disease: Juvenal referred to writer's itch (*scribendi cacoethes*) as a sick obsession (7.52).[3] At the end of his tenth satire, Juvenal added his famous plea, which might serve as a motto for all Roman satire, namely, the best one can ask for is "a sound mind in a sound body" (10.356).

In Renaissance and later *Narrenliteratur,* such as Johann Beer's *Narrenspital* (1681), foolishness was often depicted as a cancerous tumour, which insidiously overcomes ever more victims and is cured only with difficulty. It has been suggested that in the seventeenth century, art in general abandoned the demand for realistic imitation and had emphatic recourse to analogies, metaphors, hyperboles and paradoxes.[4] One expression of this changing aesthetic atmosphere was seen in the increased attention given to medical themes and images in literature and in the adoption of medical or physiological titles for books, such as Thomas Nashe's *Anatomy of Absurditie* (1589), John Donne's *Anatomy of the World* (1611) or the anonymous anatomy of a conscience, *Anatome joco-seria conscientiae* (1664). This fashion coincided with the development of scientific anatomical knowledge, which drew attention to the hidden structures of the human being; early modern anatomies were sometimes ostensibly moral works and employed the anatomy as an aggressive critical method to study vices (Hodges 1985, p. 6).[5] At the beginning of *Anatome joco-seria conscientiae* (pp. 3–4), the author apologised to doctors for intruding on their field by examining an anatomical issue, but his intention was to show how men in ecclesiastical, political, legal and medical professions disguised their true nature with different veils, mantles and a glossy skin and appealed to an apparently rational and justified action. The author proposed to perform a post mortem on a cadaverous Germany, which was releasing an ugly stench of iniquity into the world.

This anatomical act of revealing men's inner corners was a satirical act par excellence and characterised the genre not only in the seventeenth century, but also in earlier and subsequent periods. For Northrop Frye, anatomy was the synonym of Menippean satire, its most famous representative being Robert Burton's *Anatomy of Melancholy* (1621). Frye preferred to call Menippean satire anatomy, because it dissected and anatomised disabled intellectual behaviour and, in his words, the Menippean satirist saw evil and folly as diseases of the intellect (1973, pp. 309, 311).[6]

Given that medical imagery was continually used both in verse satire and in Menippean satire to discuss man's moral and intellectual existence, this study is intended to provide an introduction to medical issues and images used in the tradition of Latin satire. What kinds of diseases were satirically described? What functions had physical diseases in satires? What was the therapy? I will explore how generic conventions shaped the representations of disease, from general moral aspects to the role of the satirist and the (supposed) curative effects of satire on readers. I will focus on selected ancient and early modern Latin satires that toyed with medical topics and commented on individual immoral conditions. These texts range from morally critical satires written in the tradition of Roman verse to the more ambiguous traditions of paradoxical disease encomia. Another group of source materials includes late fifteenth- to early seventeenth-century poetics, humanist commentaries and prefaces to Roman satire that maintained a close relationship to ethical issues and considered satire as a form of healing instruction. Antonio Minturno (c. 1500–74), Jacobus Pontanus (1542–1626) and Daniel Heinsius, among others, used diagnostic and therapeutic vocabulary in their poetics when defining the satirist's duty to cure suffering and disturbed souls. The analogy was one way to defend satire from attacks against its immorality and to insist on its usefulness.

In the following pages, I will first briefly explain what I understand with the concept of medical analogy. Then I will introduce the reader to the moral nature of satire and briefly explore its relationship to moral philosophy. This is useful in showing how these two moral discourses overlapped especially in terms of their ethical goals and the medical analogies, which they frequently employed. The ancient philosophical uses of medical analogy supply clues to understanding certain details and discussions in the satirical texts, which also frequently referred to the Latin Stoics, Cicero and Seneca in particular. For example, the arguments against the grief caused by suffering were culled from ancient philosophical sources. After this introduction, I will tentatively present two issues that will appear repeatedly throughout this discussion – the figure of the physician and images of disease.

The analogy

Although my primary objective is to answer the question of how medical metaphors and terms have served satirical critique, for clarifying the background it is important to observe the use of medical discourse in different contexts. The goals of healing have traditionally been associated with all kinds of writings, not only with satires. During the Renaissance the curative effects of all poetry were often expressed in medical terms, and poetry was regarded as an instrument of moral discourse, bringing health to sick minds and driving out vice by offering virtuous and uplifting examples to imitate. Nicodemus Frischlin (1547–90), a German satirist, Protestant and professor of poetry and history at Tübingen, argued in his speech on the dignity and utility of poetry, *De dignitate et multiplici utilitate Poeseos* (1568), that poets were doctors of life who marked noble aspirations with white chalk and things to avoid with black carbon. Frischlin's interpretation of poetry, to which verse satire belonged, was clearly moralistic; in their appeals to poetry's salutary effects, other authors often also attributed this action to the beauty of the words and the sweetness of the verses rather than exclusively to the ethical content. But all stressed that the relationship between poetry and medicine was never merely metaphorical, for diseases had a psychological and physiological foundation and the healing of poetry affected both aspects of the human being (Weinberg 1961, pp. 17–23; Schmitz 1972, pp. 49–52). Other discourses, such as incantations, prayers, religious sermons, comedy,[7] love poetry[8] or consolations,[9] have also been regarded as therapeutic speech. Sophism, the art of persuading through words, was understood as verbal catharsis, and Gorgias compared persuasive speech with healing drugs (Nussbaum 1996, p. 51; Deupmann 2002, p. 95). Christ was called *Christus medicus* in medieval theology (Steiger 2005), and God was called "the celestial physician" by the church fathers and Petrarch (Carraud 2002, pp. 177, 423). However, therapeutic discourse was particularly prevalent in the Renaissance and frequently took the form of satire.

Ancient medical doctors and philosophers in particular were popular sources for ancient and early modern Latin satirists in this sense.[10] Galen (129–c. 199), whose medical thinking showed the heavy influence of philosophy, believed that the faculties of the soul were dependent on the mixtures in the body, and the mind's condition could be improved by improving physical health (Sellars 2003, pp. 67–8; Scarborough 1969, p. 115). Even though Plato is considered the first to have made the mind subject to philosophical purification or catharsis (Laín Entralgo 1970, pp. 127–37), the analogy between medicine and philosophy was more pervasive in Stoic texts than in other Hellenistic schools. Chrysippus of Soli (c. 280–204 BC) wrote at the beginning of his *Therapeutics* (his fourth book *On Affections*) that "it is not true that whereas there is an art, called medicine, concerned with the diseased body, there is no art concerned with the diseased soul, or that the latter [art] is necessarily inferior to the former in the theory and therapeutic treatment of particular cases" (trans. Tieleman 2003, p. 144). Chrysippus compared disease of the soul, which is subjected to the random motions of affections, to a feverish state of the body. The Stoics related all qualities to the body: the soul was corporeal, and thus virtue and vice also had a corporeal basis. Stoicism paralleled physical and moral sickness/wellness, and the well-being of the soul was discussed in terms of the balance of the body and the equilibrium of its humours. Health resided in a balanced proportion of the four elemental qualities in body and soul alike (Tieleman 2003, p. 157). Passions were largely understood as disturbances and harmful diseases that needed to be cured by philosophy whose rational and wise words were regarded as medicine for the disordered soul. It has often been stressed that due to the corporeality of the soul, the relationship between medicine and philosophy was not simply a decorative stylistic device in Stoic thinking, but rather good advice and learning were thought quite literally to advance moral and physical health as well (Tieleman 2003, pp. 144–7).

Cicero (106–43 BC) also discussed diseases of the soul. In the third and fourth books of *Tusculanae disputationes*, Cicero praised philosophy as therapy for the sick. He claimed that diseases of the soul were more dangerous and numerous than those of the body. He encouraged everyone to act as his own doctor, stressing in the Stoic manner the importance of self-examination in making progress towards virtue. The role of philosophy in healing was crucial (3.3.6, *Est profecto animi medicina, philosophia*).[11] Cicero claimed that it healed the soul, took away unnecessary troubles, set one free from desires and expelled fears (2.4.11). The body and the mind were sane and healthy when balanced and tranquil and when beliefs and judgements were in harmony (4.13.30). Wisdom was called a sound and healthy condition of the mind, whereas desires confused the mind and were therefore called the mind's distress or pain (*aegritudo*) or disease (*morbus*) (3.5.10).[12] They resulted from contempt for reason (4.14.31).

Seneca (5 BC–AD 65) used medical metaphors vividly, for instance, in his *Epistles*, where his own poor condition, aches and sufferings were often an excuse for his philosophical discussions, and he frequently referred to the curative function of wise words.[13] Most of the images he used were taken from the field of pathology and therapy and applied in comparisons describing the human condition and the philosopher's duty to cure suffering and disturbed souls. For example, Seneca defined hardened and chronic vices such as greed and ambition as diseases that were persistent evils and therefore difficult to control and sometimes incurable (*Epistulae* 75.11).

Among the popular ancient philosophers, Plutarch (c. 45–125) also had a special interest in medicine. His works abounded in medical references and common sense advice on good living. When dealing with virtue he claimed that "a soul possessed of excessive pain or joy or fear is like a swollen and feverish body" ("On moral virtue", *Moralia* 452A; trans. W. C. Helmbold). In another passage he compared the soul suffering from pains and outbursts of passion and anger with physical straining and convulsions ("On the control of anger", *Moralia* 457C). The moral instruction he gave for living the good life was related to physical health as well, since, as he said in "Advice about keeping well", the less expensive things were usually healthy for the body, while luxury went hand in hand with illness (*Moralia* 123D–E). Disease imagery was much used by Plutarch when defending moderation. He advised men who were living luxuriously to put a stop to their insatiate desires or else they were "but decanting wine for a man in a fever, offering honey to a bilious man, and preparing tid-bits and dainties for sufferers from colic or dysentery [...]" ("Virtue and vice", *Moralia* 101C; trans. Frank Cole Babbitt). In Plutarch's view, ailing men were not strengthened by drinks and tasty foods, but only brought nearer death. Restoring the healthy balance through an ordered lifestyle and self-restraint was also the satirist's goal.[14]

The diseases treated by philosophy were above all the diseases of belief and judgement or of passions and desires. The remedy offered by the philosopher was *logos*. The frequency of the analogy was confirmed by Cicero who took an interest in the analogy, but also complained of being tired of the excessive attention given to such over-elaborate images (*Tusc.* 4.10.23).

In the manner of philosophers, satirists have stressed the instructive function of their poetry and proclaimed themselves to be healers of individual and collective corruption. The satires that I will examine here often summarised popular ethical thinking, as mediated by the Roman Stoics, and cleverly applied its favoured themes and devices, including medical images, which had passed from philosophy into diatribe and satire. Although the philosopher's advice to restore balance in the body, for example, by adhering to a strict diet had its parallels in Hippocratic medicine's dietary regulations, it is important to observe that medical images in the satires studied here were not determined by medical developments or borrowed from medical science; rather, they continued and participated in the moralising discourses of ancient (Stoic) philosophy in which the analogy between wise words and medicine was common. Satire also affected Roman philosophy: Marcus Wilson (1997, pp. 57–8) claims that in Seneca's ironic epistle 99 ("On consolation to the bereaved") there was a marked resemblance to Roman satire; moreover, Horace's epistles had clearly influenced Seneca's epistolary practice. According to Wilson, when Seneca ridiculed his opponents he used satire as a key weapon in his rhetorical armoury. Therefore, throughout this study I will discuss how the pervasiveness of the analogy built between satirical writing and medicine reflected the influence of philosophical thinking. This shows the significance of philosophical issues and debates for the interpretation of Latin satire.

Shared goals of satire and moral philosophy

A Leipzig professor of theology, Friedrich Rappolt (1615–76), who wrote a commentary on Horace's works, was among the numerous early modern authors to note the close connections among satire, moral philosophy and medicine (1675, Caput III). By reference to Cicero and Plutarch, who both saw philosophy as therapy for the sick mind and the vices that resided either in the reason or the appetites, Rappolt attributed the same twofold function to satire (*rationis et appetitus, utriusque partis morbo, ut Philosophi, sic et Satyra medetur*). Satire cured both the intellect and the passions by driving out ignorance and purging the human appetites of bad habits. In Rappolt's view, the object of satirical pharmacy was found in the unhealthy appetites and infirmities of the mind and the reason.[15]

Renaissance poetics and humanist commentaries on Roman satire repeatedly stressed these ethically healing goals and noted the close connection between moral philosophy and satirical writing.[16] Isaac Casaubon (1559–1614), who composed an influential treatise on Greek satirical poetry and Roman satire, *De satyrica Graecorum poesi & Romanorum satira libri duo* (1605), argued that Roman satire consisted of two main principles: moral doctrine and wit (*urbanitas, sales*). Like poetry in general, satire was characterised by eloquence and the art of verse, but its main content differed from other poetry in being devoted to condemning vices and recommending virtues and using humour and jests as its tools to reach these goals (Schäfer 1992, p. 59). Satire not only set out to heal the moral and emotional life of the patient by attacking his appetites and passions, but also to cure his intellect of ignorance and foolishness. It aimed at an overall perfection of the soul, and thus the two fields of moral discourse seemed to share the same interests. The utmost healthiness of the texts was also realised in the characterisations of individual authors. Horace in particular was frequently identified as a healing satirist and his sermons equated with drugs and mixtures that medicated the sick soul of the sinner. And later Goethe claimed that the Jesuit satirist Jacob Balde (1604–68) resembled a pineapple, reminding him of all kinds of delicious fruits without, however, losing his own palatable individuality (Schäfer 1976, p. 161). The parallel activities in the fields of satire and philosophy were appreciated still in the twentieth century, as is clear from such articles as C. W. Mendell's "Satire as popular philosophy" (1920), in which satire was studied as a popular presentation of practical philosophy. But if satire did not equal moral philosophy, how did it differ from it? This question was also formulated as: how did satire deliver its criticism?

One difference often noted was that the goal of satire was to cure people of vices and false beliefs as sources of misery, but instead of offering reasonable argumentation, comprehensive doctrine or systematic theories about the good life, satires were therapeutic in a different manner.[17] As Horace put it, philosophers gave reasons why things were desirable or avoidable, but satirical moral criticism was based on illustrative, warning examples of people who exceeded the proper mean: "Invalids who are tempted to over-eat are given a fright by the funeral / of the man next door, and the terror of death compels them to go easy; / in the same way young folk are often deterred from doing wrong / by the ill repute of other people" (*Sermones* 1.4.126–9; trans. Niall Rudd). Vices that were approached as abstract concepts in philosophy were turned into concrete examples of the misdeeds and wrong actions of human beings in order to make the ethical point appealing and clear. The benefits of a frightful reflection on the dying were also recognised in the medieval tradition of the *contemptus mundi*. It recorded graphic and macabre details of death's horrors and of bodily putrefaction in order to visualise human misery (McClure 1990, p. 24).

The concrete representation of vices did not merely reinforce moral conclusions but formed the essential equipment of the genre. Casaubon claimed that:

> Roman satire shared with moral philosophy an interest in morals and manners, but these two fields had their characteristic ways of dealing with the issue. Philosophy acted by teaching; satire, mainly by condemning; the philosopher inquired into the nature and reasons for virtues and vices, whereas the satirical poet castigated the vicious and only rarely praised the virtuous.[18]

Filippo Beroaldo the Elder (1453–1505) noted that "satirists philosophised by bringing to light the secret crimes and shameful deeds of women and men and thereby restoring them to good health [...]; the satirists' censuring verses have the same effect as philosophers' books and dogmas" (quoted in Latin in Pagrot 1961, p. 55). Georg Pasch (1661–1707), a professor of practical theology and philosophy at Kiel, who discussed literature's ability to transmit morals in his *De variis modis moralia tradendi* (1707), voiced the same difference in his Preface as follows:

> When dealing with virtues and vices, historians and poets do not consider these in an abstract way (as the Logicians do); nor do they in the manner of philosophers mine their causes or nature. Instead they present men devoted to virtues or vices, assessing their deeds and manners and giving examples that are either worth imitating or avoiding. Thus, they advise us silently to watch human lives and take them as a model.[19]

Compared with satire, the philosophical teaching methods were considered dogmatic and founded upon meagre rules and sombre precepts. Thomas Farnaby (c. 1575–1647) argued in his commentary on Persius that satire added life to this dryness by drawing stimulating examples and detailed descriptions of vices. Farnaby equated satire with Aristotle's ethics and Epictetus' and Seneca's Stoic learning (1650, A2^{v}). Jacobus Pontanus concurred in his *Poeticae institutiones* (1594, p. 173), saying that:

> although satire should forcefully urge men to attain virtue and to avoid vices, it does not perform this task by arguing. Such commissions were left to philosophy, which was the sole master of virtues and an interpreter of vices. Satire required a clever, sharp-eyed, swift, eloquent and astute mind that did not abhor or abstain from playfulness.

Thus, the humanist poet Conrad Celtis (1459–1508) and his pupil Joachim Vadian (1484–1551), the latter in his *De poetica et carminis ratione*, even suggested that the teachings of Plato and Aristotle could be replaced by such satirical philosophers as Horace.[20] The German Protestants took pains to legitimise Horace's satires as the renewal of the ideal co-existence of eloquence and wisdom, considering his satires useful to Christian thinking in their ethical criticism, but rejecting their Epicurean tones (Schäfer 1976, pp. 45–52). And Frischlin claimed that reading Horace was useful to philosophers, because he presented salutary precepts of living in a much more beautiful form than Chrysippus or Crantor (1609, *Epistola dedicatoria*, p. 4).

Even though satires have usually spoken for healthy moderation and plain living without relying on specific philosophical schools or theories, the Cynic–Stoic philosophy furnished the main background of whatever identifiable philosophical content there was in classical satire. Both the ancient Cynics and the Stoics acquired the reputation of being frank preachers against the immoral. Francesco Robortello (1516–67) remarked in his treatise on satire entitled *Explicatio eorum omnium quae ad satyram pertinent* (1548), that Greek philosophers also used malediction in correcting manners. Socrates, Diogenes, Menippus, Democritus and the Cynics in general were mentioned here as the predecessors of satire (1970, p. 503). Socrates, of course, was mentioned on account of his famous irony and playful mode of argumentation, and the jocular-serious attacks on vices by the Cynic Menippus were continued in Menippean satire.[21] This satirical form was also indebted to philosophy, but in a different way than Roman verse satire. According to Casaubon, the Roman polymath Varro mixed philology and philosophy in his satires and offered healthy precepts in verse (1605, p. 259). In Casaubon's view, Varro wrote playful philosophy (p. 267, *philosophia ludens*), and Lucian also concealed serious philosophy under his comic joyfulness (p. 268). But in their Menippean satires moral issues were never addressed in a normative manner. If Roman verse satire contained serious ethical instruction under a playful cover, Menippean satire was "not merely a pleasant form for the statement of ethical truth", as Joel C. Relihan put it (1993, p. 17). Rather, Menippean satire parodied philosophical thought and discourse that aspired to express the truth in words. Thus, Menippean satire parodied satirical preaching and instruction as well. But not even in verse satire were moral norms unambiguous, since their consistent irony and exaggeration often undermined and destabilised the thesis the satirist seemed to submit. For example, Jacob Balde's satirical poetry, although written in the tradition of verse satire, expresses the Menippean tension "between jokes at the expense of philosophy and jokes in the service of philosophy" (Relihan 1993, p. 181). Thus, there were many degrees in and between mere didacticism that offered elementary ethical lessons and playfulness for dealing with moral issues in a more ambiguous manner. This attitude of *serio ludere* in exploring moral issues also suggests a certain freedom with moral standards.

The satirist as an expert healer

Of the medical images and characters used in satirical analogies, the figure of the physician was centrally important. In early modern satires the physician often played an ambivalent role, and the satirical texts balanced criticism with praise of doctors. Inept physicians were popular figures of fun in various humorous texts – Renaissance satires, epigrams, anecdotes and *facetiae* collections – that condemned the incompetence of quacks or laughed at the scatological facilities used in therapy. Doctor stereotypes were suspected of a myriad of moral failings, including plotting, poisoning, adultery, false ambitions, appetite for fame, money-making, violence, superficial diagnostics, blind reliance on book learning, lack of training, haphazard prescription of medicines and the use of incomprehensible diagnostic language redolent with Latin nonsense.[22] They were represented as the only human beings allowed to kill without punishment, even being well rewarded for their questionable services.[23] For example, Euricius Cordus (1486–1535) was a fertile German epigrammatist and a medical doctor in Bremen, whose poems fiercely attacked doctors (IJsewijn and Sacré 1998, p. 113). Heinrich Bebel's (1472–1514) three books of *Facetiae* (1508–12) contained – along with stupid peasants, lusty women, corrupted monks and other traditional sources of ridicule – amusing stories of doctors' errors familiar from the medieval exemplum tradition. One of his stories went like this (II.15, *De errore cuiusdam medici*): A certain doctor had an old and a young patient. The old but rich man was newly married to a blooming younger woman; wishing to ensure his matrimonial happiness, he asked for *diasatyrion*, a kind of Renaissance viagra, while the young patient, who suffered from fever and indigestion, was prescribed laxatives. But the doctor mistakenly mixed up the medicines, causing a most unpleasant night for both patients: the adolescent suffered from an all-night erection and the old man, embracing his bride in preparation for an erotic struggle, got diarrhoea and soiled the wedding bed with excrement.[24] Another popular anecdote recorded a similar confusion when a blind man accidently swallowed the urine and faeces that a doctor was examining for signs of illness (*Nugae venales*, p. 316; *Antidotum melancholiae*, p. 73).

In his *Medicinae gloria*, Jacob Balde, whose medical satires will be discussed below, derided the incompetence of *simiae medicorum*, female quacks and poisoners (1651, *Praefatio*, p. 368).[25] Likewise, popular collections of Latin anecdotes, epigrams and short word studies, such as *Iocorum atque seriorum centuriae* edited by Otho and Dionysius Melander (1617), *Antidotum melancholiae joco serium* (1668) and *Nugae venales* (1642), which was addressed to serious men and fathers of melancholics, printed by Nemo and published in Ubique, contained a number of medical (mainly scatological) anecdotes and invectives against unqualified healers. One popular story (*In medicum quendam*) told of a physician who was so well versed in sending men to the Underworld that his son did not need a grammarian to instruct him about the Hades myth (*Nugae venales*, p. 320). Another frequently reprinted epigram claimed that in the patient's eyes, doctors were three-faced monsters (*Aesculapius trifrons*): the first impression left was of a human being, but when the patient prayed that God or an angel would come to heal him, Satan entered, demanding burdensome remuneration (*Nugae venales*, p. 320; *Antidotum melancholiae*, p. 73). The angel, *angelus*, was also an anagram of Galenus (Wiegand 1992, p. 249).

Various discursive traditions, such as proverbs, provided further examples of doctors' suspicious work: Christian Lange (1619–62), himself a professor of physiology at Leipzig and a dean of the medical faculty, discussed in his medical miscellany, *Miscellanea curiosa medica* (1688, Ch. XXVI), the etymologies of the common proverb *mentiris ut medicus* ("you lie like a medical doctor"), which in Lange's words expressed ingratitude. Other popular and ironic sayings were the slightly modified Hippocratic aphorism *ars longa, vita brevis* (Engelhardt 1992, p. 40), and *recipe decipe*, which associated prescriptions with giving and deceiving through a phonetic likeness, as if through an incantation (*Nugae venales*, p. 10).

Such attacks and prejudices against doctors were extremely common in early modern pictorial and literary satire. But in this study I will not deal with the medical doctor as a traditional, stereotypical object of derision, but with his less familiar role, that of a rational voice and a representative of the satirical author. In Roman verse satire, the satirist often identified himself with a medical doctor who treated his patient either as a worried friend or a stern examiner. An example of the physician's role was to be found in Horace's first satire, directed against greed, where he described the lot of a wealthy man who had caught a feverish chill. Contrary to the patient's expectations, he was not surrounded by his family members preparing poultices or calling the doctor to relieve his pains, but instead his wife, son, friends and neighbours were waiting for his struggles to end in another, final way (*Sermones* 1.1.80–5). A very similar scene is found in satire 2.3. Unlike the family members, the doctor here was a loyal friend (*medicus* [...] *fidelis*, 2.3.147), as he was in Seneca's *De beneficiis* (6.16.4–5), taking personal and assiduous care of his patient in the name of humanity and compassion. For Seneca, a good doctor was present when needed, feeling his patient's pulse, advising on what to avoid and prescribing remedies. Seneca's ideal doctor was acting out of love and motivated by deeper concern for the patient's welfare; this role of a persistent guardian was taken up by the satirists as well.[26] The satirist's curative role was noted in Horace's epistle (1.1.34–5), which defined healing words as a remedy: words and sayings soothed the pain of a heart inflamed with greed and wretched craving and helped it to get rid of the ailment.

This expert position had its parallel in philosophical discourse and in the authoritative role it gave to the doctor. For example, Marcus Wilson has observed that the therapeutic metaphor used in philosophy "presupposes a physician sufficiently calm and detached to make accurate diagnoses and offer apt and salutary counsel" and "a patient whose needs are primarily negative, to obtain release from pain and illness" (1997, p. 48). This dichotomy between the healthy therapist and the sick patient also characterises satire. In the manner of a philosophical teaching situation, there was a marked asymmetry of roles: the doctor represented authority; the patient, the obedient recipient of this authority. Thus, doctors were truth-speakers, and the satirist as an ideal doctor adopted not only the expert's authoritative position but also his habit of skilful critical examination. The doctor-satirist voiced the author's professional opinion of the moral condition of man. In his *De constantia sapientis* (13.2), Seneca remarked that the wise man's attitude towards all men was like the physician's to his patients. He did not scorn touching their private parts if they were in need of medical treatment; he endured patients' insults, for he knew that all men, especially those who were well dressed in togas and in purple, were, despite their strong and wealthy appearance, unsound and similar to sick men.

In his essay entitled "Whether the affections of the soul are worse than those of the body", Plutarch remarked that diseases of the flesh were detected by the pulse, and temperatures and sudden pains confirmed their presence, but evils of the soul were more difficult to detect (*Moralia* 500E–F). They escaped the notice of most men and were therefore worse evils, since at the same time they deprived the patient of self-awareness. Only a sound reason, such as the philosopher-doctor's, could perceive the diseases, whereas a sick soul could not properly judge its own afflictions. Plutarch cited ignorance as the greatest disease of the soul, stressed the importance of self-awareness and accused mentally and morally sick people of rejecting the help offered by philosophers. And in another essay Plutarch deemed incurable those who took a hostile attitude towards admonishment and helpers; the prospects for progress were, therefore, weaker in their case ("How a man may become aware of his progress in virtue", *Moralia* 82A). Just as human beings should learn to know the peculiarities of their own pulse and to recognise pathological symptoms in their body, so in the same way they were responsible for knowing their minds and souls. Physicians assisted in the development of self-awareness, but most importantly the patient himself should take charge of his own condition (cf. Nussbaum 1996, pp. 344–5).

Roman satirists shared this view. They frequently pointed to their targets' ignorance and stupid refusal to obey the doctor's orders and to accept a much-needed remedy offered to them. In his *Epistles*, Horace marvelled that madness often went unnoticed by the patient, who nevertheless needed to have a doctor or a guardian nearby (1.1.102, *ne medici credis nec curatoris egere*). Horace argued that if someone's lungs or kidneys were attacked by an acute disease, such a person normally looked for a cure (*Epistulae* 1.6.28–9), or when he suffered from eye disease, he immediately used ointment (*Sermones* 1.5.30). The same thing should take place in dealing with moral health. Horace also described a doctor's futile attempt to cure a boy from quartan fever. Thanks to luck or the doctor, as Horace put it, the boy had already succeeded in shaking off the fever, but his mother had prayed for him and promised the gods that should he be cured, she would allow him to stand naked in the River Tiber on fasting day – with serious consequences to the patient (*Sermones* 2.3.290–5). Here Horace construed an antagonism between the religious, irrational mother and the rational healer. Superstitious men and women cast the doctor from their house and classified all diseases as afflictions of an evil spirit or a malicious god. Instead, diseases should be rationally interpreted and treated by an expert healer. Likewise, Juvenal argued that women who were ill were particularly prone to resort to astrological methods. When a woman got an itch in the corner of her eye, she used no prescribed ointment before studying her horoscope, and when sick, she followed a careful timing for taking food in accordance with the recommendations of an Egyptian priest and astrologer whom she assumed to be possessed of the utmost expertise (6.578–81).[27] William Anderson has noted that the antithesis between a wise doctor and a stupid patient appeared in Persius' satires as well, even though the doctor was more eager to point out the patients' sicknesses than to cure them (1982, p. 178).

Both in Stoic philosophy and in satire, the sick soul equalled an irrational soul. The key contrast evoked was between reason and human beliefs or desires (Cicero, *Tusc.* 3.11.24). In the manner of philosophy, satire opposed people's reliance on wishing and prayer instead of judging their condition rationally. Divine forces, gods or fortune were not to be seen as punishment for wrong deeds; rather, punishment was natural in the sense that it followed directly from bad living. The satirists spoke forcefully for personal responsibility and individual moral choice; man was to accuse himself, his sinful excesses and luxurious way of life for sickness and misfortune.[28]

The early modern doctor was still a moral instructor who acted as an advocate of abstinence and sobriety and admonished patients to shun drunkenness and control the passions. In his declamation, asking whether an orator should be preferred to a philosopher or a medical doctor (c. 1497), Filippo Beroaldo remarked that a philosopher was also a doctor, since he medicated the diseases of the mind, which were more frequent and pernicious than physical diseases (1648, p. 169). The doctor here responded that he was a philosopher of the body. In his extensive medical treatise *Institutiones medicinae*, Daniel Sennert (1572–1637) still considered these two arts to be closely related: by quoting Galen he stressed that a good physician should be well instructed both in medicine and in philosophy (1628, p. 132, *si quis optimus Medicus est, eundem esse Philosophum*). The philosopher, the satirist and the medical doctor all emphasised moderation and self-restraint as conducive to health. Plutarch said that a man recovering from an illness is satisfied with plain bread, cheese and cress. The convalescent luxuriated in little, and in Plutarch's words this was the condition in which reason reigned in the soul ("Virtue and vice", *Moralia* 101C–D). All the professions claimed to see through their respective objects and penetrate into the private sphere of great men. In the manner of the physician, the satirist examined the patient scientifically and gave advice for good living. The phases of diagnostics, from description to conclusion, were equivalent. Medicine and satire both adjudicated between the normal and the pathological, while satire also made moral diagnostics by separating the innocent from the guilty.

This cathartic process and the art of separating the good from the bad also became an important technical instrument in the early modern discussions of the goals of satirical writing. In Chapter 2, "Medical Meta-language", I will deal with Daniel Heinsius's ideas and those of his followers (especially Giovanni Volpi) about satirical catharsis. Heinsius became famous for his argument that satire had purifying effects on its readers similar to those of tragedy. The purging effect was thought to contribute to the reader's moral improvement. Although Heinsius's ideas of satirical purging became a commonplace that has often been mentioned in earlier histories of satire, in order to show the deeper relevance of the analogy I will examine in more detail his conception of satirical catharsis and the emotions of hatred, indignation and laughter that were essential in this purifying process.

However, in his *Cankered Muse*, Alvin Kernan has noted in studying Renaissance satire that at times the doctor-satirist abandoned his role as a good man and turned into a sadistic and malevolent quack, who tortured his victim and finally killed him, not for love of virtue or for the sake of healing, but for punishment and just for the fun of doing so (1959, pp. 93, 194–8). Such satirical attacks were difficult to justify by appealing to moral motives. At the end of Chapter 2, I will briefly deal with some sixteenth-century polemical satires, in which the traditional therapeutic images were reworked to punish the sins of specific contemporary enemies. The punishments took the form of therapeutic suffering, evident in such satires as Nicodemus Frischlin's anti-Catholic reactions against a certain convert Jacob Rabe (c. 1567–68) and in the anonymous Reformation satire *Eccius dedolatus* (1520).

Internally sick: appetites as diseases

Different discourses conceptualise diseases disparately. In Christian rhetoric, diseases were often conceived as being a consequence of the Fall of Man or as evidence of divine reactions against either communal or individual sin (Siraisi 1990, pp. 4–10). Illnesses were interpreted as spiritual trials that the sufferer should patiently accept. Disease metaphors have also been used to represent evil forces spreading through society. For example, the rhetoric of gouty swelling was used to depict the spread of wars, riots and other social disorders (Porter and Rousseau 1998, pp. 216–28). The world at its worst has been called a madhouse or bedlam (Engelhardt 1992, p. 40; Blanchard 1995, p. 43).[29] The suggested decay of the state has been described with diseases that punished whole communities or by arguing that an epidemic, like a laxative, purged the body politic of its waste products and criminals (Tomarken 1990, p. 92). Apocalyptic satires have recorded signs indicating the end of the world, including famine, diseases, catastrophes, wars and the movements of the Turks. Epidemics also created circumstances that were useful in testing people's morals. For example, Nathan Chytraeus's (1543–98) hexameter poem on the plague, *Contra pestem epistola satyrica* (1578), recorded the horrors in Rostock during a plague, showing how men's civility degenerated in a state of emergency. The plague as a mass disease released anarchic tendencies in the social order and disguised people's fundamental selfishness and animalistic natures in the same manner as, for example, Thucydides, who had described the effects of the plague in his *Peloponnesian War*. Chytraeus's poem disclosed the discrepancy between ideal humanity and social reality burgeoning with crowds of swine-like men (Kühlmann 1992; Kemper 1987, pp. 105–17).

Later Balde suggested in his *Medicinae gloria* (1651, *sat.* 3) that a sign of the golden age when Saturn reigned supreme was that there were no doctors and no need for their profession either, since diseases did not trouble men until Jupiter became an alcoholic; with this god's addiction and his subsequent hangover, the battalions of aches and diseases spread in the world. Consequently, men began to medicate themselves with different exotic drugs, such as asses' ears, whales' sperm, crocodiles' droppings, putrid liquor squeezed out of glow-worms, and frogs' entrails mixed with the rotten viscera of ravens. Balde pointed out that during the golden age men were satisfied with apples and water – simple and healthy nourishment that not only kept the doctor away, but also reflected men's unspoilt virtue. Modern hydrophobia was a pathological sign.[30] Balde's descriptions presumably derived from Seneca's claim (*Epistulae* 95.15–18) that degeneration manifested itself in the birth of complex and unaccountable diseases resulting from high living.

However, my focus is not on the social satire that addressed a plurality or entire societies, but on ethical satires that spoke to the individual patient and externalised his inner perversion in diseases. Although

Juvenal mentioned that the corruption of society spread like a plague and one bad apple spoilt the bunch (2.78–81), in general the emphasis was on the wellbeing of each individual. The texts studied for this project can be called introspective in the sense that they emphasised a retreat within in the Stoic manner and self-examination as a way of finding true life. Aristotle (384–322 BC) noted in his *Nicomachean Ethics* (1097a) in comparing ethics with medicine that a doctor cured individuals, and as in moral philosophy, the medical arguments in the Latin satires studied here concerned the health of a single person, not primarily of a community. Their means to cure were not to be sought from the outside, but in the patient's own moral improvement. As Cicero put it in his *Tusculanae disputationes* (3.3.6) when describing philosophy as a medical art of the soul, we must endeavour with all our strength to become capable of doctoring ourselves.

In the texts studied here, the patent symptoms of diseases and signs of imbalance in the patient's body were interpreted and treated as symptomatic of his hidden confusion. The internal disorder manifested itself in ulcers, nausea or a swollen and inflamed state that Cicero compared with the sick imbalance of anger (*Tusc.* 3.9.19). Among the favourite physical diseases and symptoms encountered in satires in general were queasiness in the stomach and indigestion (indicating luxury and other moral disorders), fever (representing passions) and gout (stemming from indulgence). The diseases were usually annoying and harmful (such as scabies or black bile); they tended to become chronic and were often incurable (such as gout), but were usually not directly lethal.[31] The satirists maintained that such disorders never had strictly physical – or supernatural – causes, for the physical condition was part of a wider moral system. As Plutarch put it, "disease grows in the body through Nature, vice and depravity in the soul are first the soul's own doing, and then its affliction" ("Whether the affections of the soul are worse than those of the body", *Moralia* 500C; trans. W. C. Helmbold). In all moral discourse it was always worse to be sick in soul than in body, but these conditions were interdependent.

Thus, in the satires studied here health and disease were considered in terms of balance and imbalance, as they were viewed in Hippocratic medicine. Although in the seventeenth century the body was perceived as a machine and sickness was explained as a form of mechanical breakdown, early modern Latin satires still maintained old ideas presented about disease in traditional humoral pathology and ancient philosophy. Disease was largely regarded as the outcome of poor diet, personal misbehaviour and faulty lifestyle.

In Stoic philosophy, passions and disturbances of the mind were connected with an unhealthy desire that never left a patient in peace once it attacked. Cicero quoted Ennius, saying that a sick soul never ceased to desire (*Tusc.* 3.3.5, *aeger* [...] *cupere numquam desinit*). Likewise in Roman satire, the sick soul suffered from insatiate hunger for luxury, excessive drinking, sexual abandon and feverish desire for fame and money. Medical discourse was used in this sense, for instance, in Horace's satire, where he equated human vices with mental illnesses and offered the traditional ancient medicament, the biggest dose of hellebore to the greedy (2.3.80–2). Greed and avarice were regarded as particularly persistent and hardened illnesses, which made the patient pursue women, wine or money, if there was no reason to settle and cure the desire. Horace noted that a man who suffered from fear or desire was unable to enjoy his wealth, because sore eyes have no pleasure from seeing beautiful pictures, nor aching ears from music (*Epistulae* 1.2.52–3). Cicero spoke about avarice, the keen desire for money, as being an evil that circulated in the veins and diseases ensued (*Tusc.* 4.11.24). Thus, the medicament needed to be given in large doses.

Desires that had become excessive were not addressed in satires as abstract appetites but literally and directly; the human body became the incarnation of vices, as in the old Attic comedy in which the parasite had been merely a belly or Terence's Gnatho was mere jaws. Satires centred the reader's attention on the glutton's swollen stomach, saliva adhering on the lips[32] and his mouth opened wide to yawn (implying sloth) or to swallow large mouthfuls: "We lift wide our jaws and regale with grin and gape" (Lucilius 3, frg. 131; trans. E. H. Warmington). The word used here of the mouth is *rictus*, which is mainly applicable to wild animals. In his late fifteenth-century commentary on Horace's satires Christoforo Landino (1424–98) interpreted the open mouth either as a sign of avarice and vehement desire or of sick inertia and laziness (1486, *ad loc.* Hor. *sat.* 1.1.71). Gluttony and uncontrolled appetite for power were turned into concrete images in Seneca's moral discourse as well: Antonius was likened to a giant maw engulfing Pompey's property, and the contemporary world was likened to an all-consuming and swollen stomach (Gowers 1993, p. 19), which became an image of moral aberration in Roman satire. The word used for the stomach was often *abdomen*, more properly associated with pigs' stomachs and suggesting man's bestial qualities. Persius' poems in particular had a strong emphasis on physical images. In his verses bad poets prayed for a hundred mouths, tongues and throats with which to recite their bombastic verses more loudly (5.1–6); and the throat, a metaphor of avidity, was used meaningfully in the plural (3.89, *fauces*), as was observed by Renaissance commentators (Britannicus 1613b, p. 76, *fauces* [...] *summum gulae, eaeque numero tantum plurali*).

Violent impulses were particularly suitable for moral discourse, which called for control of reason. Satires showed the consequences of the pathological condition in which the body led the mind. As Horace put it, "the body, / heavy from yesterday's guzzling, drags down the soul / and nails to the earth a particle of the divine spirit" (*Sermones* 2.2.77–9; trans. Niall Rudd).[33] This condition when the soul was moist from too much drinking – as the scholiast explained the phrase – not only harmed its capabilities, but human beings also became slaves to their own unlimited appetites; their body parts were turned into autonomous entities that made constant demands and had a life of their own. Exhortations to free the mind from its slavery to the body were commonplaces in Seneca's moral epistles as well (14.2; 65.21).

Persius made a comment on random living by blaming a lazy student for neglecting to notice where his legs carried him (3.62). In the same way, in ancient philosophical discussions the empowering effect of intense passions, which took hold of men and carried them away, was sometimes compared to running legs, which cannot be controlled in the way that walking can (Braund and Gill 1997, p. 9). In Juvenal's ironic words the starving stomach (*ventris furor*) forced the cannibal to gnaw his companion's bones (15.100–2). In another passage the belly gone mad made independent decisions and swallowed the silverware, the cattle and finally, the whole farm in order to satiate itself (11.40–1). In the same way women's insatiable sex organs forced them to continuous love-making against their will and without reasoning (6.129; Miller 1998, p. 265). With these hyperboles Juvenal underlined the need to take responsibility for one's life and for the rational control of appetites based on physical requirements. In his *De medicina*, Celsus had also spoken ironically about people who, in justifying their desires, blamed their perfectly innocent stomachs, finding fault in the weakness of the stomach instead of in the will (1.8.2). The conclusion was that the body as such was not to be accused as being the primary source of delusion and appetites, but rather the mind, which did not control its desires, was the culprit.

Hidden wounds and symptomatic colours in Roman satire

Since the Roman satirists established the imagery of disease as an essential part of the satirical tradition, I will briefly deal with a few specific pathological symptoms found in their verses. Medical motifs were important in constructing moral criticism in Roman satire, in which all physical symptoms conveyed moral values and were metonymical in the sense that they raised larger issues about the human condition. The body was nearly always discussed in negative terms (cf. Miller 1998), as a site for moral illnesses, and the condition was expressed in the language of pathology. Disease metaphors dominated Persius' first and third satires and showed up in several Horatian passages.[34] Medieval and Renaissance commentaries on Roman satire already paid critical attention to these terms and images, as well as to the concept of disease. In their commentary on Juvenal (first edition 1498), Antonius Mancinellus and Jodocus Badius Ascensius noted that *morbus* referred to the overall corrupted condition of the body, *aegrotatio* added infirmity to the disease, and *vitium* implied a discord in the agency of the body parts, which caused their deformity (1515, xix^{v}–xx^{r}). Johannes Britannicus mentioned in his commentary on Juvenal's satires (first edition 1501) that *morbus* was an acute infirmity of the body, whereas *vitium* was its permanent deficiency (1613a, p. 56).

One of the pervasive features of all satire is that it studies forms of deception and draws attention to pretense, hypocrisy, self-deception and other vices that have discrepancies between appearance and reality. As Juvenal noted, "never have faith in the front" (2.8).[35] Discrepancy was also revealed through the use of medical diagnostic terms: Horace memorably introduced Lucilius as the first "to draw back the glossy skin" when exposing pretensions of the rich and powerful (*Sermones* 2.1.64–5).[36] Satirists were expert examiners who sought to remove the white toga or the glossy skin, to see behind the deceptive appearances and reveal the rottenness and soreness within. Among the satirical metaphors developed from medical and physical terms, skin was one of the central images for a surface covering that disguised recesses and inner perversion (Bramble 1974, p. 153). The skin was often given such attributes as glossy, greasy, attractive and shining; these ironic qualifiers highlighted the false impression left by the outer appearance.[37] The same falsifying function was attributed to an oil-rub (4.33), which made the skin shine, and to suntan, since taking the sun was perceived as a vain attempt to hide the true colour: "What's your idea of the highest good? To dine for ever / among the flesh-pots and pamper your skin with regular sunshine?" (Persius 4.17–18; trans. Niall Rudd). A French philologist Nicolas Rigault (1571–1654), among others, observed in his commentary on Juvenal (10.192) that the word used for the skin was often *pellis* (instead of *cutis*), which means animal skin or the skin of a corpse, thus further degrading the target (1684, *ad loc.*). Moreover, the word *pellis* was often used in conjunction with *intus* or *introrsum*, and the inside was defined as ugly or shameful (*turpis*), even though it glittered outwardly. The skin not only indicated "skin-deep", but became a metaphor for basic character as well. Persius noted in his fifth satire how *pellicula* (a disparaging diminutive for skin), that is, the wrapping, once acquired was difficult to cast aside. People were born within the skin in which they remained throughout their satirical lives: "You retain / the skin of your old disguise and wear a glossy exterior / while keeping a cunning fox inside your vapid heart" (5.115–17; trans. Niall Rudd). The satirist, however, emphatically claimed to know "what you are underneath, in the skin" (Persius 3.30, *ego te intus et in cute novi*).[38]

The bloated skin mentioned in Persius' third satire (3.63) has often been understood in its technical sense, and scholars have claimed that it refers to dropsy, but it is needless to attempt to ascertain the cause and nature of such symptoms or discuss them in strictly technical terms.[39] They can instead be read as supporting the poetics of satire, which construed an opposition between the inside and the outside. Tumescent skin implied that something ill was hiding inside and developing secretly to the point that it was nearly bursting out for everyone to see; "your flesh is already sick and bloated" (Persius 3.63; trans. Niall Rudd). Skin concretely covered illnesses, which then manifest symptoms on the surface: black bile accumulated in the chest, the body swelled and augured a coming attack (Persius 5.144–5). Swellings were also openly moral symptoms, suggesting ostentation, arrogance, self-importance and other disorders of the mind described by the satirists. Sometimes the swollen state was more specifically defined as madness or rage according to the humour (black bile) that caused the tumescence. For Cicero, tumescence implied perturbations of the soul, such as sadness or anger, whereas the wise man's soul never swelled with such passions (*Tusc.* 3.9.19).

Other symptoms referring to the sore inside were also diagnosed: for example, the patient's foul breath signalled internal disease. Breath (Gr. *pneuma*) was, in Hippocratic medicine, a central concept, and health was defined as the result of its free flow, whereas diseases accrued from the difficulty of digestion and the impeded passage of the pneuma. The breaths rising from undigested food were described as unhealthy vapours that caused diseases (Tieleman 2003, p. 195). Seneca too noted the significance of yesterday's fumes and belches: they indicated that the food and presumably the man were both rotting (*Epistulae* 95.25). These medico-philosophical views were shared by the satirists: Lucilius

(3, frg. 130) and Persius (3.99) both referred to sour belches arising from the chest,[40] and the patient was short of breath in Persius' satire, presumably because his heavy burden of sins made breathing freely difficult (3.89). The words *gravis halitus* referred to a bad and ominous smell. The famous passage (3.88–103) gave a vivid image of a dying man who had over-indulged in sensual pleasures. To sooth the initial symptoms (chest palpitations, sore throat and difficult breathing), the man requested a smooth Surrentine wine to drink, but the medicine only exacerbated his condition. A similar passage was found in Juvenal's first satire (1.140–6), which described a sick gourmand who failed to digest huge amounts of boar and peacock meat; a heart attack struck like lightning.

These examples suggested that the real reason for the various symptoms lay in the internal condition. The philosophers had emphasised that if illness found a place in the inner body, the more severe and inveterate it would become. In his *Epistles*, Seneca described how luxurious habits gradually penetrated the sinews of the body. The worst evil afflicting people was not external, but was situated in their very vitals and difficult to discern or cure (114.25). Cicero also claimed that the feverish excitement of the soul settles in the veins and marrows and thus becomes a chronic disease (*Tusc.* 4.10.24). Persius noted that people should therefore take care of themselves in the early stages of a disease (3.64, *venienti occurrite morbo*), before their case was hopeless; otherwise medicine would need to be particularly strong to reach the internal organs.[41] Likewise, it was necessary to realise first that one was sick in order to attain soundness. Therefore, Seneca repeatedly claimed the moralist's need to see (*inspicere*) vices and internal corruption underlying an attractive surface (*Epistulae* 115.9).

In the representation of internal evils, the image of the hidden wound was frequently used. It was a concrete and ominous detail that marked the patient, and its soreness emphasised the pain that a latent illness must cause its bearer. The wound image was used in social and political contexts to denote a corrupt society; different passions were also viewed as ulcerous sores in the self.[42] Juvenal used the wound metaphor specifically to represent hatred, "a wound that can never heal" (15.34; trans. Peter Green). Enduring a painful wound was also used to illustrate self-discipline, virtue and bravery. Enduring pain made men examples of self-mastery and, in Cicero's view, of Roman heroism and Stoic fortitude.[43] The rhetoric of military asceticism renounced pleasure and languishing in luxury and spoke instead for the hardening of the self for the rigours of life – these being represented by the image of wounds.

However, in satires the wound represented a significantly different image. It was a sign of inflammatory erosion, where healthy material was gradually reduced to rotten and putrefying flesh. In comparison with an epic, where heroes inflicted clear wounds on each other as they struggled for honour, in satires wounds were not caused by blows or cutting weapons, but arose internally. They were abscesses and boils that did not arise from heroic qualities or bestow fame; their relationship to honour was the reverse. Likewise, Seneca talked about internal sores in terms of abscesses and ulcers that were deep within his breast (68.8).[44] As in medicine, the violence and the site of the disease were crucial. In Persius' third satire, which was held together by a disease metaphor, the satirist examined his patient, a reluctant young student of philosophy who appeared superficially healthy (his pulse was steady and there were no signs of fever). But when asked to open his mouth, the patient revealed a nasty "septic ulcer at the back" (3.113–14, *latet ulcus in ore / putre*). The expression gained almost proverbial power; in form it resembled Virgil's famous saying, *latet anguis in herba*, which also referred to a latent and hidden evil (*Eclogae* 3.93). Moreover, the wound was purulent and signalled the young man's rotten condition. Again, in comparison to Seneca's words in *Consolatio ad Marciam* (1.8), wounds were easy to heal if they were still fresh. But when they hardened and had festered, they had to be cauterised, opened up and violently crushed. According to Celsus' *De medicina* as well, ulcers that passed down into the throat were dangerous, especially to children, and recovery was difficult (6.11.3). The technical verb *inspicere* used twice by Persius for the doctor's conduct (3.88–9) recalled diagnostic language; the doctor literally looked in. The inner wound was visible only to the satirist, who had the means to peer deep into the soul of the patient and then display the corporeal scene for others to see.

The wound image recurred in Persius' fourth satire (4.43–5). This time it was in the groin and covered by a broad golden belt. Here the deceptive discrepancy between the internal character and the outer appearance was highlighted by the wound's gold covering, just as inner weaknesses were often covered over by fame, money or other glittering things that put up a false front. Horace also censured the habit of fools hiding open wounds instead of discussing them with a doctor and seeking a cure (*Epistulae* 1.16.24, *stultorum incurata pudor malus ulcera celat*). Plutarch noted that inward ugliness was too often concealed as if it were an ulcerous sore; the moral progress of such a man was not likely to be significant. As a model worth emulating, Plutarch named Hippocrates the physician, who publicised his own error and failure to apprehend the facts about cranial sutures ("How a man may become aware of his progress in virtue", *Moralia* 82B–E). Similar openness in confessing and announcing one's own mistakes and shortcomings, instead of concealing them, was also expected from other human beings. The same advice was given by Philosophy in Boethius's *De consolatione philosophiae* (I.4.1, *Si operam medicantis exspectas, oportet vulnus detegas*).

A hidden wound as a symbol of inner weakness revealed by the physician-satirist was also found in Juvenal's sixth satire, which has been regarded as a quasi-medical text, *remedia uxorationis,* intended to cure Postumus, who was getting married (Wilson & Makowski 1990, p. 29). The poem described a woman who carefully made up her face with cosmetics (*medicamina*) that only created a deceptive mask: "But all these medicaments and various treatments [...] make you wonder what's underneath, a face or an ulcer" (6.471–3; trans. Peter Green). The phrase "a face or a wound" (*facies dicetur an ulcus*) epitomised the essential satirical contrast between the apparent (for the face was the body part usually visible to others) and the real.[45] The final position of the word *ulcus* underlined that in order to see the true essence one had to dig deeper. In Juvenal's second satire (2.11–13), the physician-satirist showed similar visual acuity. He examined the shaven lower parts of a man who had concealed his homosexuality under a virile and bearded (and thus philosophical) appearance. Although the visible parts left an impression of a real man full of vigour – symbolised by the shaggy hair, just like the mythical heroes Heracles and Polyphemus – the patient had a hidden physical condition, haemorrhoids, in the secret area of the anus.[46] This condition resulted from anal sex, as the physician laughingly discovered before he began to burn the haemorrhoids away. Thus, there was hardly any private sanctum into which the satirist's gaze did not penetrate to uncover the hidden nature of human beings. By looking into the sore and private corners of his patient, the satirist uncovered hidden blemishes and exposed them for everyone to see and censure. In addition to exercising their power in this way, satirists liked to think of themselves as transgressors of conventional boundaries, with the skin marking a critical border that they crossed. The wise man himself was, of course, invulnerable.

Paleness was another common symptom that clearly indicated some latent illness that insidiously gnawed and tormented the body and anticipated an approaching condition of lifelessness. According to medical literature, paleness often resulted from some infirmity in the stomach (Celsus, *De medicina* 1.8.2). In Horace's satires, the reason for paleness was attributed to over-eating: a man was "pale and bloated from gluttony" and after a heavy meal, sticky phlegm rebelled in the green-looking diner's interior (2.2.21, 75–7). In Persius' satires as well, the words *pallor* and *pallere* frequently appeared as bad omens of forthcoming sickness and indicators of general indisposition.[47] For example, the man who died while bathing after an undigested meal had a white stomach (3.98, *albus venter*).[48] A memorable example of paleness was also found in Juvenal's first satire, where a man earning his inheritance in a rich matron's bed "looks as pale as the man who steps barefoot on a snake" (1.43; trans. Peter Green); here paleness indicated sexual excess and the young man's reluctance to perform this labour. Often passions and disorders, such as a bad conscience, fear or love-sickness, appeared on the human surface as pallor (Bramble 1974, pp. 148–51). Money and the worries it induced were represented by cool colours, too: Horace used the verb *pallere* in his accounts of the curse of ambition and the morbid love of money (*Sermones* 2.3.78). Persius' satires used the same word with an explicit reference to money and avidity (4.47, *viso si palles, improbe, nummo*). Cornutus noted in Persius' satires that the satirist himself was trained to scrape away pale (that is, sick) behaviour (5.15).

Thus, a pale physical appearance was a qualitative symptom and involuntary manifestation that once again reflected and indicated the inner condition. It was not a mere physical reaction, but also a cognitive and moral symptom related to the patient's moral character. Horace defined pallor further as guiltiness (*Epistulae* 1.1.61, *pallescere culpa*). In addition to foretelling a poor prognosis, it reminded of the patient's past actions: it was a later-symptom that succeeded some offence or crime that the person had committed. It was the colour of fear and the accused and stemmed from shameful deeds and their coming to consciousness (cf. Martial, *Epigrammata* 2.24, *pallidiorque reo*, "paler than the accused"). Juvenal described how guilty men "blanch and tremble at every lightning-flash", referring to guilt, which made people regard every bad symptom as a punishment sent by the gods (13.223, 229–32).

Juvenal also mentioned sweating – the alteration between cold and warm, fear and shame – as a physical symptom of guilt (1.166–7); Rigault interpreted the alteration as signifying a bad conscience (1684, *ad loc*).[49] The author of *Rhetorica ad Herennium* already noted that our changing colours, paleness and blushing, are symptomatic of our conscience and attend either guilt or innocence (2.5.8).[50] Plutarch also argued that man's body was affected by the impulses of his passions and this "is proved by his paleness and blushing" ("On moral virtue", *Moralia* 451A; trans. W. C. Helmbold). He illuminated the knowledge of one's dreadful deeds and personal errors by the image of an ulcer as well, saying that bad conscience "leaves behind it in the soul regret which ever continues to wound and prick it" ("On tranquillity of mind", *Moralia* 476F; trans. W. C. Helmbold). Regret together with shame were persistent ulcers, since they were caused by reason that chastised itself in the feeling of disgrace.

The change of colour was usually seen on the face, that is, the site attacked by the satirists. Hippocratic medicine, for example, advised to pay special attention to the patient's facial appearance and look for any changes produced in the face by long or severe sickness. This pathological *facies Hippocratica* was characterised, for example, by sunken eyes and cold ears.[51] However, the image of inside paleness offered by Persius pointed directly to the real site of the disease (3.42–3, *intus / palleat infelix*). Blushing and paleness spread on the face but, in Seneca's words, these conditions in fact arose from the depths (*Epistulae* 11.1). In the sense of moral guilt, the symptom of paleness was so common that Martial constructed a paradox with it. In Martial's epigram (1.77), Charinus was chronically pale, although he was healthy, drank moderately and had good digestion. Still, paleness indicated moral defects, for Charinus was pale even after having rouged his skin and while licking someone's ass. The point was that he did not know how to blush, that is, he was not innocent.

It is thus important to observe how medical terms were used in constructing moral criticism in Roman verse satire. Medical terms and the analogy between diseases and vices were used in ancient moral criticism to the extent that in Horace's satire (2.3) such discourse was ironically placed in the mouth of a funny convert, the Stoic Damasippus. In another passage (2.4), Horace played on the conventional didacticism by offering a parody of gastronomic lectures for healthy living. Nevertheless, medical images became a firm and conventional part of the tradition. In the later literature the arguments against bad living were often taken from Roman satire and its images of wounds and paleness recurred, for example, in Renaissance poetics and in satires written against drunkenness and other vices.

Changing traditions: from rotten insides to disease encomia

In the tradition of Latin satire diseases were often emblems of the human immoral condition. In Chapter 2, the focus is on poetics and the reception of Roman verse satire, including late fifteenth- to early seventeenth-century poetics and other discussions of the genre, which repeatedly applied the medical analogy to characterise satire and emphasise its healing function. But in my work as well as in the Latin satirical tradition diseases were at times also more positively assessed. In Chapter 3, "Painfully Happy", I endeavour to broaden the view of satirical moral criticism by focusing on early modern disease eulogies, which were produced especially in Germany, Italy, France and the Netherlands. In these texts, harmful diseases and physical deformities were no longer represented in terms of imbalance or confusion of the mind, but instead were praised as useful, beneficial and even beautiful. In her *The Smile of Truth* (1990) Annette H. Tomarken has illuminated the multifaceted satirical encomium with emphasis on the sixteenth-century French tradition, and in his *Scholar's Bedlam* (1995) W. Scott Blanchard has identified the mock encomium as an enormously popular rhetorical form and an important subgenre of Renaissance Menippean satire (pp. 15–16). However, in her work on Neo-Latin Menippean satire, Ingrid De Smet (1996, pp. 74–5) argues that the paradoxical encomium does not belong to the genre of Menippean satire, since it is non-narrative and does not have a plot structure. Instead, it must be seen as a form of epideictic oratory. If we agree with her strict definition, then the early modern eulogies of fever, gout and the itch studied here – as being non-narrative prose works and essays without any fantastic setting or prosimetrum – do not belong to Menippean satire. But on the other hand their playfulness and lightness of touch when dealing with moral and philosophical issues and their frequent use of paradoxes clearly connect them to the Menippean traditions.

In such eulogies, the conventional assumptions about disease were questioned by redefining the concept. In his *Podagrae encomium* (c. 1546), Girolamo Cardano (Hieronymus Cardanus, 1501–76), who held the chair of medicine in Pavia, argued that gout was a disease only if disease were defined in terms of pain, but not if the prerequisites for something being a disease were mental and physical languor, folly, desire, lack of awareness of the human condition, anger or sadness (1619, p. 218). For Cardano, the gravest diseases were those of the mind. But the negativity of disease was also questioned by claiming that many renowned poets and intellectuals had suffered from different diseases: Virgil from melancholy, Lucretius from insanity, Ovid from stupidity (!) and Horace from inebriation – and yet they had been famous and productive men. Besides, man's divine origin became visible when he was ill: he was able to foresee the future, contemplate serious matters and be free of the perturbations of the mind. Even incurable diseases, which for Seneca had been a sufficient justification for suicide (Colish 1985, p. 49), were viewed as a benefit that greatly increased the quality of life. The patient who was forced to stay at home could devote himself to private study and agreeable detachment. He was forcibly alienated from physical passions and vanities that normally surrounded him in his daily life and that diverted him from the good and gradually led to vice.

The paradoxical encomium spread widely as an oral and literary genre in the Renaissance, culminating in Erasmus's *Encomium moriae* and continuing well into the later seventeenth century. Lucian's satirical dialogues and praises of a parasite, of a fly and of gout were important in disseminating the tradition (Marsh 1998; Robinson 1979). During seventeenth-century polyhistorism, everything in nature was thought to be full of the wonder of divine creation, and the largest anthologies of paradoxical encomia emerged during that century. The most extensive anthology was Caspar Dornau's (1577–1631) *Amphitheatrum sapientiae Socraticae joco-seriae* in two volumes (1619). Dornau's compilation includes hundreds of praises and shorter descriptions excerpted from larger works. Not all of these are paradoxical or satirical texts, but it also included serious praises and non-literary, medico-botanical studies of diseases, plants and animals. Dornau explained the mention of Socrates' name in his title as a reference to a playful way of philosophising and questioning false opinions, which often had recourse to praises of things that the multitude held as being of little value (Seidel 1994, p. 350; Tomarken 1990, pp. 51–2). The second volume by Dornau – who himself was a medical doctor and a philosopher – assembles praises of vices and diseases discussed below, including fever, gout and blindness.[52] Shorter but equally popular and often reprinted collections were, for example, *Facetiae facetiarum* (1615); *Nugae venales* (1642); *Dissertationum ludicrarum et amoenitatum scriptores varii* (1644) and *Admiranda rerum admirabilium encomia* (1666). The latter contained nearly thirty playful eulogies of animals and diseases (cf. Appendix).

I will examine how the disease encomia relied on philosophical and Stoic ideas about pain, suffering and disease and how these philosophical discussions were structured in the satirical paradox form. By this approach, I wish to enhance understanding of the suggested philosophical and medical aspects of satirical criticism.

Chapter 4, "Wonderfully Unaware", continues with satirical Neo-Latin disease eulogies but focuses especially on physical features that somehow affect the intellect, namely, the sensory disabilities of blindness and deafness, and somnolence. These eulogies were often consolatory, dedicated to friends (formerly) active in politics or in education and now suffering from some chronic disability, and meant to comfort them and furnish strength in their suffering. Satirical playfulness, consolatory rhetoric and philosophical wisdom were combined here. In philosophical literature, the *consolatio* was considered a vehicle for therapy of the emotions; hence, the consolation has been called "the paradigmatic instance of the therapeutic mode of philosophising" (Wilson 1997, p. 48). Likewise, the eulogies playfully reminded one that for a wise and virtuous man contentment was possible in any circumstances. Authors like Jacob Guther (1568–1638) alleged that the opinion of Everyman about blindness being a misfortune was misleading, since wisdom did not require eyes if the mind was illuminated nor did the disability deprive men of anything essential to their happiness. On the contrary, blindness and deafness protected men from the evils of the world. The suffering body was no longer a negative affliction of the soul, a burden or a necessity that connected the human being to the animal world, thereby necessarily separating him from the divine spheres, but rather a physical ailment paradoxically released the soul from its chains. All the texts examined here are from the late sixteenth- and early seventeenth centuries, including the eulogies on blindness by Jacob Guther, Jean Passerat and Erycius Puteanus, the little-known praise of deafness by Marten Schoock and the praise of somnolence by Christoph Hegendorff. These texts were also often reprinted in the playful Renaissance anthologies of ironic encomia. In the fourth chapter I will also deal briefly with drunkenness, one of the most popular vices in Renaissance satires. In Roman satire wine never scattered troubles or gave consolation to or relief from suffering, as it did in convivial poetry. Rather it was a motif that reminded humans of their mortality in a different way, not by encouraging them to take pleasure in the moment, but by showing how drinkers lost their health and were no longer able to seize the moment, even if they wanted to. But in the Renaissance encomia drunkenness was now also welcomed as being conducive to the overall sanity of the body and the mind.

The final chapter of this book, "Outlook and Virtue," further illuminates the use of medical and physiological images in Latin satire by focusing on descriptions of hilariously imaginary illnesses and various forms of physical ugliness. It shows how very different physical functions and peculiarities acquired moral qualities. Thus, it dwells on a playful speech about dwarfs (by Albert Wichgreve) and on poems about the morally acceptable outlook of virtuous and intellectual men, including the characteristics of extreme thinness and ugliness of philosophers and poets (in Balde's satirical poetry). The physical deformity that generally provided material for making jokes was now extolled as useful and beautiful. The chapter also deals with a number of pseudo-scientific mock dissertations and treatises on imaginary venereal diseases of first-year university students, *beani* and *pennales*, and considers theses on unusual ailments that turned young men into rabbits (*De hasione*). These texts took their inspiration from student humour and learned university discussions. Mock dissertations followed the usual structure of academic disputation and its devices of pedantry, listing, categorising and quoting authorities, but instead of analysing serious scientific issues, these dissertations were full of vulgar, scatological jokes and dealt with something commonly regarded as trivial or vicious, such as sexual abandon or the intriguing question of whether "a fart had a corporeal or a spiritual basis". The treatment of such afflictions was harsh and violent, and in addition to the conventional hellebore, more imaginary medicaments, heavy drinking or flatulent dishes were recommended. It is also worthy of note that sometimes the patients were Stoic philosophers and intellectuals, authorities otherwise held in esteem in moral satire.

The purpose of this final chapter is to show how different and even eccentric physical features could be morally interpreted. It also offers an appreciation of the variety of Neo-Latin satire and its carnivalistic and morally ambiguous tendencies. Pseudo-scientific treatises or anatomies of a medical topic are an important and sometimes neglected part of the tradition. Günter Hess, for example, in his otherwise thorough study of German Renaissance literature of folly, saw that the sixteenth-century *facetiae* collections marked a degeneration of satire and a trivialisation of its comic devices (1971, pp. 240–1). His assessment does not do full justice to the texts that may not be refined in humour but nevertheless were frequently reprinted and thus apparently were popular reading among academic youth. These satires reacted playfully to their former moral criticism, reusing traditional satirical images and calling into question moral stereotypes that had earlier been advocated as valuable. By vividly describing moral failings such as diseases but without any moralistic instruction, these texts also parodied the earlier satirical tradition and its preaching tone and amused the audience rather than communicating doctrine or stabilising values. Thus these texts can be seen as representing the traditions of Menippean satire, which makes jokes at the expense of learning and calls into question all value systems, philosophical doctrines and the moral certainties of verse satire. Disease images were transformed to serve mere amusement or the criticism of morally critical discourse itself.

2
Medical Meta-language: Renaissance Commentaries and Poetics on the Healing Nature of Satire

Although the Roman satirists emphasised their curative role and identified themselves with doctors, they did not use medical images as persistently as their Renaissance counterparts. This does not mean that the medical analogy would have been forgotten in the Middle Ages; on the contrary, medieval authors and commentaries on Roman satire also drew attention to medical terms (Witke 1970, p. 188; Kindermann 1978, pp. 60–3). But it has been stated that in sixteenth-century theoretical statements on satire, the genre's functions, methods and nature were expressed almost exclusively in medical terms, which did not occur in any other genre. Furthermore, Mary Claire Randolph proposed that this imagery went out of fashion later, in the seventeenth and eighteenth centuries, when vices were no longer characterised as ulcers but as ruling passions that needed to be tempered by reason and judgement rather than healed by a physician-satirist (1941, pp. 125–6). Rationalistic terminology replaced the physical terms that had been common in earlier Renaissance discussions of satire. It was thus in the sixteenth- and early seventeenth-century theoretical works on satire that the medical task was most widely acknowledged. In this Chapter, I will take a closer look at this Renaissance commonplace about satire's therapeutic function.[1]

Medicine as a metaphor for writing satire

Among the Renaissance poetics, Antonio Sebastiano Minturno's (c. 1500–74) *De poeta* (1559) contained a famous passage on the parallel roles of medicine and satire:

> Diseases and ulcers of the body are the material of medicine on which it entirely concentrates, whereas satirical poetry has focused on the diseases of the mind (*morbi animi*), which can be called its subject matter. Both fields endeavour to improve health, of the body and of the soul, respectively. As the means of cure, the one uses drugs, the other, words; one offers bitter drinks, the other, severe reproof. Philosophy is medicine for disturbed souls and the philosopher takes care of curing vices as well, but unlike the philosopher, the satirist does not deal with virtues, but with issues that are called the opposite. The satirist wittily, humorously and not without indignation censures vices in verse in order to mend people's manners. (1970, pp. 423–4)

The same imagery reappeared in Minturno's Italian treatise *L'Arte poetica* (1563).[2] Minturno's views had a strong influence on English Renaissance literature. The idea that satires advocated a homeopathic healing method using purges has been seen as due to his influence (Pagrot 1961, p. 75). However, in the use of the medical analogy, Minturno was preceded by Cristoforo Landino, who in the preface to his commentary on Horace's oeuvre in 1482, referred to the medicinal nature of the author's satires and epistles. Landino noted that Horace called his satires *sermones* in order not to frighten the reader away from their salubrious content. Landino attributed to these *sermones* the philosophical task of purging the human mind of decay and informing men of the best morals (*ad mentes humanas olim labe purgandas & optimis moribus informandas*). He stressed that Horace's doctrine equalled in usefulness the majority of philosophical books (1486, cxvii). Satirical instruction was needed because most people were in a pathological condition: they were naturally weak-minded and enervated or else wrong education had turned them soft and spineless. According to Landino's diagnosis, the reasoning power of a sick man was effectively dormant (*consopita ratione*) or completely buried, and therefore the appetites reigned supreme (cxvii).

Another early Italian scholar to comment on the medical nature of satire was Angelo Poliziano (1454–94). In his lectures on Persius (*In Persium praelectio*) delivered in Florence in 1484–85, Poliziano claimed that, due to our serious sickness (*gravis animi morbus*) and lack of proper self knowledge, our pathological condition often goes unnoticed by us, as if we were patients whose legs were numb, not aching, and who hence falsely regarded the absence of pain as a sign of health (1613, p. 107 [137]). Poliziano reminded us that someone nearing his end hardly felt any pain, but this certainly did not indicate good health. He recalled how surgeons had successfully used iron to resuscitate and reanimate even half-dead people and aroused or restored their forces. Encouraged by this example, men should trust their minds to satirical doctors who supervised and treated the moral condition. Such doctors completely rooted out all blemishes (*labes*), diseases (*pestis*) and seeds of disorder (*perturbationum semina*) by using the traditional means of iron and fire (*ferro et flammis*). Landino had recommended the same therapy, defending the satirists from accusations of cruelty by saying that they used fire and iron – the surgical knife – to heal wounds only in the most difficult cases, when other remedies had failed, and it was impossible to avoid having recourse to a physician's care (1486, cxvii).

From the Italian soil the medical discussions, which defended the usefulness of satire, spread to the North. A very successful poetological treatise was written in the sixteenth century by a Jesuit priest and gymnasium director in Augsburg, Jacobus Pontanus (Jakob Spanmüller, 1542–1626). Pontanus adopted the by-now familiar medical analogy in his *Poeticae institutiones*:[3]

> It is reasonable to submit the diseases of the mind to satirical criticism, because the sickness of the mind concerns the art of satire just as pains, ulcers and sick bodies concern the art of medicine. Both these arts propose sanity as their goal. One uses words; the other, mixtures and herbs. Both prepare bitter, unsweetened and distasteful medicines for patients; they operate surgically and burn the flesh, without pity. (1594, pp. 171–2, *Argumenta, finis, utilitas satyrae*)

Several times Pontanus argued that satirists should imitate physicians, especially in the use of bitter but salubrious medicine. Intellectual history has preserved many passages with references to bitter but truthful words as medical potions. Plato compared philosophy with medicine and rhetoric with flattery. In his essay "How to tell a flatterer from a friend", Plutarch stressed that at times friends needed to abandon exalting, gladdening and flattering words and instead have recourse to reproof and frankness. This frankness (Gr. *parrhesia*) was compared to a bitter and pungent-smelling medical potion mixed of castor, hellebore or a medicinal plant called *polium*, which the patient was made to drink for his benefit (*Moralia* 55A–B).

The flatterer acted in the opposite way. If a man hesitated to bathe or eat for health reasons, then the flatterer approved of the man's deceitful desires and did nothing to restrain him from his pleasures, as a friend would have done. Instead, the flatterer encouraged the man "not to maltreat his body by forced abstinence" ("How to tell a flatterer from a friend", *Moralia* 62A; trans. Frank Cole Babbitt). At the end of his essay, Plutarch, however, remarked that the dose given to a friend should not be thoroughly permeated by bitterness. Here, again, the example of the physicians was to be followed: Just as after a surgical operation the physician treated the suffering part with soothing lotions, in the same way frank speech should be mollified by gentle words (74D). Another famous dictum describing the poet-philosopher's beverages was found in Lucretius' *De rerum natura* (1.936–50; 4.11–25), where in a memorable way he offered his curative verses to readers, as a doctor sugars a healthy potion with honey.

This therapeutic and persuasive activity had its literary counterpart in satirical admonishment, which also offered bitter medicines for sick souls. The image was seen in Horace's first satire (1.1.25), where teachers offered biscuits to children to coax them to learn. In Boethius's *De consolatione philosophiae* the personified Philosophy repeatedly promised to offer harsher remedies to the patient, although she never used them.[4] Landino, Minturno and Pontanus all employed the *locus classicus* from Lucretius and Horace, repeating that the sick soul resembled a child who refused to listen to adults' admonishments.[5] The purpose of satirical humour and wit was to sweeten the brim of a glass so that the patient would not recognise the bitterness of an unpleasant medicine before it touched the bottom of his stomach. The bitterness referred to the salubrious content of the words and their biting frankness, useful but at times disturbing and frightening in their satirical language, which vividly portrayed the number and dangerous effects of vices. For Lucretius, the honey had meant the poetic form, which covered the philosophical content; here the sweetening was humour, verbal wit and the fictitious examples used to illustrate the ethical issues.

These examples help us to imagine how widely medical analogies in satirical writing were adopted by early modern authors. Jacob Balde, the seventeenth-century satirist and also a Jesuit, who knew Pontanus's poetics well, noted in his satire *Medicinae gloria* that "following the example of the author [Horace] who offered sweet cookies to patients and spiced with the bees' liquor his bitter potion, we also mix in this book such diverse ingredients as absinth and honey, juice and biting vinegar" (1651, *sat.* 1). Balde thus characterised his stylistic choices by reference to the ancient analogy. He also emphasised the healing nature of his satirical poetry in the preface to his poems:

> I will exhibit the fearless art of writing that may be something new in our age. It is akin to medicine, which abolishes diseases of the body by using bitter but efficient drinks and seasons them with sweet juices so that they would not be rejected. Satire penetrates the mind and, by removing vices, endeavours to restore the temperance of manners. Therefore, poetry would appear horrid and frightening, unless the vividly running, chill water created by Pegasus' hoofs that easily makes the reader's teeth chatter had a touch of honey obtained from Helicon. (1651, *Ad candidum Lectorem*, p. 369)[6]

In *De studio poetico* Balde claimed that although satirists collected their words and expressions from the butcher shop (meaning that their words were harsh and crude), the shop itself was situated in the Roman Forum, and the meal was lavish, consisting of acid tastes, rustic cabbages, meat and sarcasms sprinkled with sweet dew (1658b, pp. 47–8). The flavouring also included a jar of pure salt, vinegar and mustard. These ingredients – salt and mustard – were often mentioned in medical literature among the purgatives, which were used for inducing a vomit. Balde proposed in the first poem of his *Medicinae gloria* that even if he could not heal like Persius, he would still write like Matho, composing lamentations at people's graves (1651, *sat.* 1). When he defended the art of satire in his *De studio poetico*, he also used the conventional healing verbs of *sanare* and *urere* (1658b, p. 47). Although Balde boasted of the novelty of his method, he expressed the function of his satirical poetry in words that, already in the previous century, had become commonplace.

These general remarks on the healing nature of satire were often accompanied by further discussions on individual satirists as healers. Thomas Drant, an Archdeacon of Lewes in the sixteenth century, translated a group of Horatian satires in 1566, giving them the title "A MEDICINABLE Morall, that is, the two Bookes of Horace's Satyres" (Randolph 1941, p. 143; Pagrot 1961, p. 81). The edition was also prefaced with the motto *Antidoti salutaris amaror* ("the salutary bitterness of a salutary antidote"). In Renaissance commentaries, the primary purpose of Persius' satires was seen as being the castigation of human vices and making people sane (*sanus*). Federicus Cerutus (b. 1541) wrote in a dedication attached to his explanatory paraphrase of Persius in 1597 that:

> just as physicians are occupied in purging and curing wounds and bodily illnesses, likewise there has to be a way to treat – as if with

> healthy medicine – human minds suffering from vices. And even if this therapeutic effort does not turn out to be completely successful, nevertheless patients should at times be punched by biting words and at times persuaded by festive laughter to avoid wrong deeds.[7]

These examples are but a few of many that show the continued emphasis placed on satire's role as curative writing. The medical metaphor recurred not only in poetics but also in commentaries about individual writers.

The healing doctor and the sick doctor

Early modern discussions of Roman satire often made critical comparisons among the three Roman satirists, especially Horace and Juvenal, who were considered significantly different in tone and in their reasons for writing (Brummack 1971, pp. 312–20). Authors such as Daniel Heinsius and John Dryden saw that the purpose of healing was central to Horace's satires, a goal absent from Juvenal's more aggressive writing. In Heinsius's view, Horace used indirect means of teaching virtue, and his satires followed the same ironic method that Socrates had used in correcting men with false beliefs.

Whereas Horace gently healed his patients by stressing the value of simple living, Juvenal wrote in terms that suggested his own sick condition. Instead of representing him as a healer, Heinsius argued that Juvenal's satires vomited black bile (1629a, p. 172). Balde spoke of Juvenal's indignant verses, which were foaming like an epileptic; Balde doubted whether, considering the manners of his times, his contemporary authors had sufficient spleen and black bile to censure its evils and imitate Juvenal. Balde expressed his predilection for playfulness rather than for bloody and serious criticism (1651, p. 369). Likewise, in his *De ludicra dictione* (1658), the French Jesuit Franciscus Vavassor (François Vavasseur, 1601–81) remarked that Horace influenced the mind in a gentle and playful way, Persius was ironic and philosophic, but Juvenal's satires were crude and nauseating in their indignation; the author was queasy and so was his reader (Ch. 2.7, *De Horatio, Persio, Iuvenali*).[8] The vomiting associated with Juvenal was a form of involuntary physical purgation and concrete evacuation; the author could only throw up when encountering the corrupted world. Thus, the satirical purging was not a pleasurable event for any of the participants.

A similar distinction between Horace and Juvenal was drawn by the Dutch scholar Petrus Cunaeus (1586–1638) in his two speeches entitled

In Horatium and *In Juvenalem*.[9] Here, Horace was described as an author who revealed people's whip-scarred backsides and disclosed their true faces behind their illusory masks, allowing no one to remain hidden beneath an alien skin (1674a, pp. 225–6). Juvenal, on the other hand, not only attacked vices that were ridiculous (that is, moderate and bearable), but also censured serious improbity and actual crimes, which deserved to be violently punished and lanced (1674b, p. 244). In his essay *De satira Juvenalis* (c. 1616), Nicolas Rigault examined Juvenal's fiery style and argued that Juvenal had armed himself with a horrible whip with which, burning with indignation, he painfully lashed worthless people.[10]

Despite his sadistic aggression, Juvenal was not a mere executioner. Rigault saw him along with the other Roman satirists as a philosopher through satire. In Rigault's view, stylistic differences among the three satirists were caused by their differing historical contexts. In the deepening degeneration of imperial Rome, the satirists gradually needed to adopt a more severe attitude and disavow the role of physician in order to be heard, to surpass their predecessors and to counter the increase in contemporary corruption. In contrast to the happier times under Emperor Augustus, laughter was forbidden during the reigns of Nero and Domitian. In Rigault's lively description, the involuntary suppression of laughter set off a physical reaction in Juvenal. The restrained laughter first changed to indignation and pain, then gradually grew worse and finally turned to anger, leaving the impression that the poet was on fire within (*velut aestuantibus praecordiis*). This condition, which does not escape flatulent associations, was reflected in Juvenal's passionate style and in his manner of chasing people's vices with the already familiar instruments of iron and fire (*ferro flammaque*).

The Roman satirists themselves often also appealed to a kind of a bodily urge and compulsory physical need that was pressing their innards and making them write satire. Persius said that he was unable to rule his spleen (1.12, *petulanti splene*); Juvenal noted that anger boiled in his dry liver (1.45, *siccum iecur ardeat ira*). Writing was a form of personal and physical release. Some modern scholars have argued that self-purgation was in fact the main function of traditional verse satire (Birney 1973, pp. 4, 13). However, the reactions that Horace's satires elicited from the reader were considered significantly different: Pontanus praised Horace for successfully playing around the diaphragm, that is, the soul of men (1594, p. 173). When sweetly titillating the reader's diaphragm, which, in Johannes Murmellius's words, was the most sensitive part of the human body, Horace's writing aroused the most pleasurable feelings (1516, xiiii^{v}).

To return to Rigault's discussion in *De satira Juvenalis*, he followed his description of the satirists with an interesting account of the physico-pathological state of Domitian's Rome. Rigault's words are quoted here in full in order to show his rhetorical vigour:

> Juvenal wrote in an age that was thoroughly contaminated by the emperors' crimes. Laws were abandoned and the government's voice fell silent. Once virtuous Rome was now degenerating and gradually falling into a state of enervation and nearly lethal lethargy (*sopore paene letali*). In awakening lethargic patients, doctors instruct to burn crude pitch, fresh wools, onions, galbanum and other substances that exude unpleasant smells, which make the patient sneeze and thus to shake his head. Likewise, satirists have to light their torches, bring them close to people, burn stinking taverns and obscene brothels and profitably illuminate the Neronian nights. Thereby, the dirt which is put into motion strikes the nostrils and the brain, and the lethargic languor (*somniculosus ille marcor*) which had overcome the Roman minds is dispersed by fierce indignation, as if by a sneeze. (1684, unpaginated)

Satire was here compared with the burning of all kinds of fumigants, and the ensuing smoke was then thought to dispel moral ills, since it made the mind purge itself and recover its consciousness as if by sneezing. The therapy recommended here echoes Celsus' advice to burn similar drugs in order to promote sneezing and to cure men of acute and lethal lethargy (*De medicina* 3.20.1–2). The benefits of sneezing were also observed in Renaissance medicine. In his *Institutiones medicinae*, Daniel Sennert stated that pepper and hellebore not only irritated the nostrils, but also usefully stimulated the brain while causing the patient to sneeze (1628, pp. 966–7, 1151). Substances that excited sneezing were called *sternutatoria*; they were particularly strong and efficient in dispersing even stagnated fluids. Galbanum, the medicament mentioned in Rigault's text, was an aromatic gum resin, which was also used as a spice. According to Pliny the Elder, the very touch of it mixed with oil of spondylium was sufficient to kill a serpent (*Naturalis historia* 24.13.21–2). Satirists were thus advised to use strong remedies indeed, and the act of cleansing taking place by the fumigations was itself a means of traditional catharsis.

Renaissance writers often expressed their predilection for either of the two moral authors, Horace or Juvenal. Among the most notable writers on poetics, J. C. Scaliger (1484–1558) favoured Juvenal in his *Poetices libri septem* (1561) and considered Persius' poems needlessly abstruse, asking what sense did it make to attempt to amend people's manners if such incomprehensible language was used that no one understood (III, caput XCVII, *Satyra*). In his *De satyrae Latinae natura & ratione* (1744, p. 115), a literary scholar and philologist from Padua, Giovanni Antonio Volpi (Johannes Vulpius, 1686–1766) argued against Scaliger's high estimation of Juvenal by claiming that:

> in amending the habits of sinners (*peccantium morbis emendandis*) it was useless to burn with fire, to adopt a threatening pose or act like a public executioner, when the purpose after all was to cure sinful patients of their diseases. Sweet and mild remedies were more efficient than caustic and irritating means in curing the diseases of the mind (*morbi animorum*). The latter way merely exacerbated the condition and day by day turned the situation to the worse, so that finally no hope of sanity remained.

In his *Discourse concerning the original and progress of satire* (1693), John Dryden, for his part, described the two Latin authors as follows:

> And let the *Manes* of Juvenal forgive me if I say that this way of Horace was the best for amending manners, as it is the most difficult. His was an *ense rescindendum*; but that of Horace was a pleasant cure, with all the limbs preserved entire; and as our mountebanks tell us in their bills, without keeping the patient within doors for a day. What they promise only, Horace has effectually performed. Yet I contradict not the proposition which I formerly advanced: Juvenal's times required a more painful kind of operation [...]. (1968, p. 138)

Between the lines Dryden was also criticising the medical practitioners of his time. The medical imagery was further elaborated on a few pages later, where Dryden derided readers who did not appreciate the value of good literature (Horace's satires) or penetrate its deeper truths, which would have given them moral sanity and happiness:

> They who endeavour not to correct themselves according to so exact a model, are just like the patients who have open before them a book of admirable receipts for their diseases, and please themselves with reading it, without comprehending the nature of the remedies, or how to apply them to their cure. (1968, p. 141)

Horace was here emphatically introduced as a doctor, but Juvenal had a different effect on his clients. Still, Dryden greatly appreciated Juvenal's mastery, and when comparing it with his satires' truncated form in translations, Dryden again used the violent physical (if not directly medical) image: "Yet there is still a vast difference betwixt the slovenly butchering of a man, and the fineness of a stroke that separates the head from the body, and leaves it standing in its place" (1968, p. 137). Medical and body metaphors were thus applied to describe the differences among the satirists, their original texts and the translations. In his preface to *Absalom and Architophel* (1681), Dryden also used the above metaphor, saying that satire endeavoured to amend vices by correction like a physician who prescribed strong remedies for an inveterate disease. This was done to prevent the surgeon's amputation of an *ense rescindendum* that Dryden did not wish even on his worst enemies (Pagrot 1961, p. 149). In Juvenal's satires the victim was decapitated as though he had been in battle.

The point made by several early modern authors in comparing Horace and Juvenal was that Horace's more pleasant, humorous and indirect way of writing satires resembled the work of a medical doctor, but in Juvenal's times more bitter medicine or even verbal execution was needed. Therefore, his satires turned to outright violence, punishing the victim and causing extreme physical pain rather than healing.

Heinsius and Volpi on satirical catharsis

In sixteenth- and seventeenth-century poetics, the satirist's violent intervention was described in surgical terms or justified by referring to satire's purifying purpose. Usually, satire was discussed in terms of medical purging (*purgatio*). Contemporary medical literature made distinctions between different forms of purging; catharsis in the strict sense meant concrete evacuation of humours through vomiting or taking laxatives (Sennert 1628, p. 1108, *purgatio in specie humorum excrementitiorum per alvum & vomitum per cathartica evacuationem significat*). However, in poetics the discussions were related to the powerful position that Aristotle's *Poetics* and the concept of catharsis had acquired in these centuries, both having become "an established pillar of a pedagogic concept of poetic art" (Meter 1984, pp. 29–30). Along with tragedy, attention was now drawn more systematically to other literary genres, and their poetics received new impetus through the application of Aristotelian concepts. Francesco Robortello was one of the famous sixteenth-century Italian commentators on Aristotle's *Poetics* – his commentary appeared in Florence in 1548. Robortello wrote poetics of comedy, elegy, epigram and satire as well (Meter 1984, p. 108).[11] By following the analogy of tragedy, scholars now endeavoured to find a similar explanation for the effects on the reader caused by other literary genres. Comedy, for example, was said to produce relief from anxiety, sadness, tension, violent aggression and even envy.[12] The idea of laughter as a remedy against melancholy was commonplace in prefaces to all kinds of comic narratives, *facetiae* collections and parodical eulogies. For example, a collection of anecdotes entitled *Antidotum melancholiae joco serium* (1668) and addressed to baron Nemo or Niemandt von Nirgendshausen, offered according to its preface "a useful antidote to melancholy that was pernicious to everyone, and turned away, repelled and repulsed the evil from individual households and doors, from thresholds and hearts, from breast and brain, indeed from the entire microcosm". However, melancholy was never mentioned as the object of satirical catharsis, but only of the other forms of comical literature.[13]

In the sixteenth and seventeenth centuries, the satiric theory was modified and modelled after the cathartic effects of tragedy proposed by Aristotle. Satirical purging was influentially defined by Daniel Heinsius in his book on Horatian satire, *De satyra Horatiana libri duo* (1612, extended edition 1629). Heinsius had dealt with tragic purgation or expiation of passions in his *De tragoediae constitutione* in 1611. For him, catharsis was the principal objective of tragedy. He regarded catharsis as a means of moral instruction and not merely as an aesthetic effect (1643, pp. 10–11).[14] The concept encompassed the medical and therapeutic meanings given to it in the philosophy of Pythagoras, which Heinsius knew through Iamblichus' *On the Pythagorean Life*. Heinsius compared tragic catharsis to the purification achieved through bloodletting, the use of emetics and vomiting by which harmful substances and fluids were expelled and removed from the body. However, he did not view such catharsis as an elimination of all the emotions, which was the Stoic interpretation, but only of the detrimental elements and excesses so that the passions and emotions were diminished to the right degree and balanced in the mind so that they obeyed reason, as prescribed by Aristotle or Pythagoras. Heinsius thus understood tragic catharsis as moderation rather than as an extirpation of the passions (Meter 1984, pp. 168–9).

After having dealt with tragic catharsis, Heinsius applied the idea to satire as well. His overall interest in the theory of literary genres and Aristotelian literary theory was probably stimulated by Robortello's studies (Meter 1984, p. 108), but the discussion of satirical catharsis was more of his own elaboration. Heinsius's definition of satire, modelled upon Aristotle's definition of tragedy, was to become famous:

> Satire is a type of poetry without a sequence of actions, and it was invented to cleanse human minds. It describes human vices, ignorance and errors and all other things, which follow from these vices in every man. It uses representation that is sometimes dramatic, sometimes simply narrative, sometimes consisting of both of these manners of representation. It often presents its criticism indirectly under a veil, using figurative language. Its style is low and ordinary, partly sharp and biting, partly witty and playful. It elicits hatred, indignation or laughter. (1629a, p. 54)[15]

The definition pointed out that the satirists employed different representational devices and various style levels. The first line of the quotation shows that satires focused on the qualities of its characters in contrast to tragedy, which imitated action and had a strong emphasis on the plot structure. However, of crucial interest here is the notion that the target of satirical writing was the human mind and its vices and that the genre's goal was purging, *expiatio* or *purgatio*. The religious-ethical word *expiatio* concerned the cleansing of sins rather than of the emotions, and it was thus very apt to be used to satirical effect.[16] Heinsius explained that the act of cleansing immoral habits was needed before the mind could attain moral consummation and true virtue (1629a, p. 55). Thus, the ethical task and moral value already emphasised by the Roman satirists and other earlier authors received an influential theoretical affirmation here, where satire was defined as a means of moral instruction through purgation.

In studying Heinsius's literary criticism, J. H. Meter has noted that for Heinsius, satirical purging was analogous to tragic catharsis; it was not "an elimination of harmful emotions but [...] the creation of an emotional equilibrium, which is characteristic of the emotional state of the rational man" (1984, p. 280). However, it is more precise to argue that even though Heinsius regarded an emotional equilibrium as the goal of satirical writing, he also noted the variety of satirical methods and their respective purposes.

Some satirists endeavoured to remove passions and emotions completely instead of moderating their harmful excess. This difference was demonstrated when Heinsius dealt with the ancient Pythagorean, Socratic and Stoic schools and their peculiar purifying methods (1629a, pp. 55–60). The first one, the Pythagorean way of purging, was mild and gentle. It never had recourse to direct attacks against passions or vices; nor did it insist on their total or immediate expulsion, because this would only have strengthened them. Instead, the Pythagorean way aspired to attain gradual improvement and reduction of the passions. As an outstanding example of this therapeutic method, Heinsius mentioned the precepts of soberness and rational balance offered by Ofellus, the wise peasant in Horace's satire (2.2), who has often been regarded as a Stoic. Yet according to Heinsius, the peasant did not belong to the Stoic or any other philosophical school. He was an uneducated rustic fellow whose virtue was based on simple living in the countryside, considered the "virtuous milieu" in Roman satire. The objective of the Pythagorean method was a rational balance achieved by gradual moderation of the passions.

The second way of purging men of their vices followed the homeopathic principle of *similia similibus curantur* (p. 59). This method too was rather gentle and used mild reprimand only. In order to correct serious vices, it did not directly set out to expel them from the soul, but offered less dangerous passions with which to replace them. A patient suffering from love-sickness or other undesirable passions was healed by exposing him to similar emotions and directing his attention to other, more acceptable objects of those emotions. Strong addictions were cured by showing the patient the true forms of love and wealth as they were understood by Plato and Socrates.

The third, Stoic way of purging applied stronger and less tolerant means for achieving virtue (p. 60). In Heinsius's words, the Stoics did not accept even minor vices or passions, which others regarded as healthy in some measure. The Stoics intended to extirpate all vices completely, applying a method called *a contrario*. Among the Roman satirists, the Stoic Persius represented this type of purging. As for the severity of the method, Juvenal would also fit the category well, although Heinsius does not mention him here. Thus the three forms of purging represented different attitudes to vices, and the three methods were thought to have their specific representatives among the Roman satirists: Horace purged the mind as did the Pythagoreans, gently and with sweet laughter, whereas Persius (and Juvenal) represented the less flexible school of the Stoics and were indignant and intolerant toward all vices and passions.

Heinsius's ideas of satirical purgation were adopted and developed further by many authors. Dryden quoted Heinsius's definition of satire and noted that the purpose of satire was to purge the minds and the passions (1968, p. 143). Ben Jonson's remarks on poetry, tragedy and satire were largely culled from earlier Italian authors and Heinsius (Sellin 1968, pp. 147–63).[17] Friedrich Rappolt (1675, Caput I–II) and Georg Pasch (1707, Caput III, §6) both quoted Heinsius's definition of satire and presented the three philosophical methods of purification. Among the treatises by later followers, *Liber de satyrae Latinae natura & ratione* (1744) by Giovanni Antonio Volpi is particularly illuminating about the purifying goals of satire. Volpi based his writing almost word for word on Heinsius, taking Heinsius's definition of satire as his starting point, but extending the discussion and adding some remarks of his own.

Volpi took into consideration Horace's exemplary figures, like Ofellus – a man content with simple living who had no objection to pleasure as such but recommended moderation. Volpi mentioned Ofellus in discussing the Pythagorean method of purging and noted that by blaming and moderating pleasure, Ofellus made pleasure more rewarding (p. 16). Volpi regarded this attitude as a direct continuation of the ancient physicians' practice and principle of healing physical illnesses called *paullo minus* intended to improve the patient's condition gradually, step by step. In Volpi's view, Horace made use of Ofellus' words in the same way as Plato owed much to Socrates' wisdom. Ofellus' nickname, *abnormis*, meant "self-taught" and suggested that he did not base his precepts on doctrines learned at school or through formal philosophy (p. 17).

In addition to Ofellus, Heinsius and Volpi also mentioned Horace's father as a simple and virtuous man of the rustic Roman past, whose moral example deserved to be followed and who had taught Horace how to censure vices with humour. Volpi maintained the idea of the excellence of the native Roman moral tradition, which was handed down from father to son and generally called *mos maiorum*. For Volpi, the virtue of simple living and popular wisdom stemming from common sense characterised Roman society as a whole, in contrast to the Greek world, whose wisdom he saw as consisting of futile words, loquacious precepts for healthy living and quarrelling philosophical schools (p. 18). The Roman discipline, although robust and uncultured, represented solidity and virtuous simplicity. It manifested itself in deeds rather than words, as with the Spartans. This opinion Volpi supported with a quotation from Quintilian (*Institutio oratoria* 12.2.30), according to which the Greeks abounded in precepts, the Romans in examples. Teaching by example was here seen as characteristic not only of the Romans but also of the Roman genre of satire.

Volpi's discussion reflected the earlier biases against the Greek culture, which were already expressed by the Roman satirists and especially by Juvenal, who had attacked everything (including slaves, music, language and clothing) that originated in Greece or abroad. As has repeatedly been argued, the Roman satirists were hostile to Greek influences, which helped them to articulate their own poetic processes and establish themselves as true and free-speaking Roman voices (Mayer 2005, p. 146). This essential Romanness of the satiric genre was thus emphasised as late as the eighteenth century through the idea that the Romans were not only more truthful and frank but also morally purified versions of the Greeks. Roman virtue was thought to manifest itself in the genre of satire. Volpi's attitude also reflects a certain anti-scholasticism similar to earlier Renaissance humanists; Petrarch, for example, had rejected loquacious scholastic philosophy by reminding that the true purpose of philosophy was to heal the human mind (McClure 1990, p. 47).

It is no surprise to discover that Heinsius viewed ignorance as one of the main objects of satirical purification. Heinsius (1629a, p. 64) and Volpi (1744, pp. 27–8) further specified two types of ignorance, through which they defined the satirical object in more detail. In the first kind of ignorance, men based their behaviour on false opinions, which thus led to wrong actions. This view of ignorance reflected ancient philosophical thought. Plato had called folly and mindlessness, which included ignorance, diseases of the soul (*Timaeus* 86b; Tieleman 2003, p. 188). Both the Stoic and Epicurean theories criticised misguided beliefs about the proper goals of human life and called false opinions diseases (Braund and Gill 1997, p. 10). The second type of ignorance was unawareness of all basic principles, a type characteristic of the common, unlettered folk and apparently the result of their poor and insufficient education; this kind of ignorance was almost non-existent among the educated. What is important according to Volpi, is that satires did not ridicule the second kind of ignorance, but usually avoided laughing at simple folk. It is a well-known fact that satirical laughter is very often directed at those in high social positions and those presumed to be corrupted by political or social power; this bias can also be seen in Volpi's primitive ideals and theorisings about satire. The ignorance ridiculed in satire thus belonged to the first type and was characteristic of the educated and well-to-do in particular; they were pseudo-philosophers and futile poets who pretended to know more than they did.

When dealing with the Socratic method of purging, Volpi (p. 21) repeated Heinsius's ideas that illnesses were cured by using drugs and remedies that resembled the sickness itself, *a similibus ad similia*. Likewise, in preventing and rejecting passions, Socrates had recommended a cure that was closely akin to the vices themselves. Therefore, for example, he acted like a lover in order to draw young men's thoughts away from dangerous and injurious forms of love. Volpi insisted that the Socratic method of correcting manners was pleasurable and sweet, caused no pain and had the remarkable advantage that patients obeyed it willingly. Unfortunately, Socrates' philosophical method of teaching morals was misunderstood by his contemporaries, and he was compelled to commit suicide for being guilty of pederasty.[18]

Heinsius and Volpi preferred the Pythagorean and Socratic manners of purging to Stoicism. Volpi regarded Stoicism as excessively severe and unconditional, since it did not tolerate any passions and made no distinctions among vices and sins, but censured all equally, be it adultery, homicide, slander or lying (p. 22). Furthermore, in his view, people lost their humanity by following Stoic rigour. By appealing to "wiser" philosophical traditions, Volpi insisted that emotions were not diseases or deemed to be futile. In addition to the Stoics' categorical thinking, he disapproved of "Epicurean softness", which in his view also exceeded healthy moderation. Volpi noted that Horace had ridiculed both these philosophical schools: the Stoics in the figures of the slaves Damasippus (in satire 2.3) and Davus (2.7), the Epicureans in Catius (2.4). For Volpi, the true and simple wisdom of the Romans was to be preferred to the affected learning and precepts offered by the Greek philosophical sects. Heinsius and Volpi concluded that Horace in particular (as well as Plato in his second *Alcibiades*) followed a successful method in teaching men how to live well when warning them about the wrong ways of living. Heinsius (p. 61) quoted Horace's words in his fourth satire, which referred to the example given by his virtuous father ("My good father gave me the habit; to warn me off / he used to point out various vices by citing examples", 1.4.105–6; trans. Niall Rudd), and another passage from the same poem (1.4.126–9), both of which emphasised the usefulness for satire of warning examples. According to Heinsius and Volpi, these excerpts revealed the essence of satirical writing, which worked through warning and fear.

Satirical effects and emotions

In satire, arousing emotions was just as important as controlling them, because the purification of the vices actually took place by appealing to certain emotions. The poetics of Minturno, Robortello, Heinsius and Volpi all maintained that the emotions universal to satirical catharsis were significantly different from the tragic emotions of fear and pity. Heinsius claimed that satire produced three specific emotions (*affectus*): hatred (*odium*), indignation (*indignatio*) and laughter (*risus*). Hatred was directed towards mean individuals or vices in general that were represented in satires (1629a, p. 73). The audience was then expected to observe the relationship between the fictional objects of hatred and the real world and to transfer the emotion towards real, sinful people. Volpi too argued (pp. 13, 42) that hatred was felt for vices or crimes and bad human beings, for example, on witnessing an attack against innocent people or seeing good men becoming victims of slander. Hatred was a basic reaction to an unjust world order. Thus, Heinsius and Volpi maintained the view of emotions that Aristotle had taught in his *Rhetoric*; the readers' emotional reactions were aligned with ethical judgements and these reactions should be ethically appropriate to the specific situation.

Indignation then means that men feel annoyed by the grief of good men, vices in general or more specifically by the success of those who do not deserve their prosperity. This feeling was very common in satire; it was both generated by satire and also mentioned as the chief cause and the driving force for writing, as Juvenal memorably put it. According to Heinsius (1629a, p. 74), indignation was easy to provoke, since people were bound to feel sick on seeing men without merit succeed. Heinsius considered indignation more difficult to bear than any other emotion. Indignation was mixed with envy if a man's social position was lower than that of men who were undeservingly overrated.[19]

Interestingly, both these negative emotions and modes of judgement seemed to be connected with the feeling of injustice. Satire described people who had succeeded unfairly; it was a reaction against such injustice. Heinsius (1629a, p. 73) and Volpi (1744, pp. 13, 42) used the Greek word *nemesis* here, meaning righteous indignation at undeserved good fortune. Aristotle had used the expression in his *Rhetoric* (1386b–87b), "a feeling of pain at someone who appears to be succeeding undeservedly"; he considered it to be the opposite of pity, which was pain at undeserved misfortune. Indignation also differs from envy, which is pain felt at others' success, but does not require that the success be undeserved. Thus, Heinsius's and Volpi's understanding of indignation was closely Aristotelian, with indignation related to an assessment of fairness and justice.[20] As such, the emotion was relevant to satirical criticism, which assesses good and bad action, and, as if in a courtroom, is intended to arouse justified and thus virtuous moral indignation among members of the audience against the guilty.

The third emotion inspired by satire was laughter, which was discussed in the context of the effects of satirical styles and emotions. Laughter, of course, characterised comedy, and Heinsius and Volpi viewed laughter as a joyful and festive form of vituperation. Horrible things did not usually provoke laughter, whereas adultery was one of its typical objects (Volpi 1744, p. 29). Satires, however, sometimes offended against this convention: Volpi considered cannibalism to be an improper subject of laughter, even though Juvenal had dealt with it in his fifteenth satire (pp. 25–6). Likewise, Rappolt noted that beastly vices like incest and patricide belonged to tragedy, not satire. He also mentioned Juvenal's poem on cannibalism as an exceptional theme among satires (1675, Caput III). Volpi argued that laughter altered the audience's mood from seriousness to hilarity so that a clear change took place in their emotions. Secondly, laughter was a remedy directed against the sad feelings of hatred and indignation that satire had earlier released (p. 13).

To clarify their ideas about laughter, Heinsius (1629a, p. 74) and Volpi (1744, pp. 44–5) divided them into two types. A bitter laughter (*amarus*) blamed and ameliorated immoral habits and was mixed with and stirred up by indignation. The second type, ridicule (*ridiculus*), acted as a solace and a remedy to the very indignation. Thus, it appears that satire first raised and stimulated specific negative emotions, exposing a reader to their excess, until they reached a saturation point, and then relieved them by the more pleasurable emotion of laughter, exactly as was thought to happen to the emotions of pity and fear in tragedy. As harmful vices that were mentioned among the diseases of the soul that satire should cure were hatred and indignation, neither of which could be the end result of the process if the genre's purpose was moral improvement. Laughter was thus needed to mitigate disturbing emotions, which were produced during the satirical experience, and restore the equilibrium in the human mind. Hence laughter was an important means for these harmful emotions to undergo the morally instructive process of purging. The negative emotions satire caused were at once the objects and agents of satirical catharsis, but laughter dominated in the end.

The issue of laughter was frequently addressed in Renaissance discussions of satire. Robortello, for example, dealt with it in discussing the nature and goals of satire in his treatise *Explicatio eorum omnium quae ad satyram pertinent* (1548).[21] Robortello's thinking was strongly influenced by Aristotle's poetics, and this heritage was reflected, for example, in the emphasis given to imitation as the basic principle of all poetry. Satire and comedy imitated human actions by using joking and laughter. Robortello argued (1970, p. 501) that laughter was caused by things that had ugliness (*turpitudo*)[22] or something wrong with them (*vitii species*). These did not necessarily cause just laughter, but could also arouse hatred (*odium*). Hatred consisted of severe reproof and did not include any sense of amusement. It differed from mockery (*irrisio*), which was laughter mixed with contempt. Satirical subjects were capable of arousing both emotions, since some types of ugliness deserved to be responded to with hatred, others with laughter.[23]

Reference to different kinds of laughter made it possible to draw a distinction between satire and other genres. Satirical (or any) laughter was impeded by events and characters for whom we feel sorrow. Robortello argued that we do not laugh at suffering people, but rather feel pity; this is the effect caused by tragedy. Likewise, horrible things gave rise to fear, not to laughter (1970, p. 501). In his *Poeticae institutiones*, Pontanus explicitly distinguished satire from tragedy on the basis of satire's subject matter, which was an ugliness that evoked either laughter or hatred, depending on which the vices deserved (1594, p. 171). Sadness, fear and commiseration had no place in satire, but belonged to tragedy.

It is important to note that Pontanus not only named the emotions proper to satire in order to differentiate it from tragedy, but also clearly stated that precisely the tragic emotions, especially pity as a form of compassion, were excluded from satire, in which no pity was shown its objects. Pity contained an impulse to approach, terror an impulse to retreat (Bennett 1981b, p. 208), but in satire men laughed and attacked from a distance. It is not by accident that the satirists were so often depicted as physicians, for rationality and a certain insensitive distance were characteristic of both. In his *De tragoediae constitutione*, Heinsius interestingly gave an example of a physician, a surgeon and a veteran soldier as men who had learned to master their feelings through habit and exercise, and this mastery enabled them to practice their professions. Heinsius remarked that "when a physician visits a patient for the first time, he is intensely affected until habit tempers his emotional response and makes way for professional competence" (1643, p. 12; trans. Meter 1984, p. 171). Likewise, anyone who repeatedly witnessed misery and horrifying events gradually became less intensely affected by them, became hardened to the vicissitudes of life and thus acquired a proper balance of the emotions.[24] The same effect could be attributed to satire, which made calm veterans out of timid recruits in the process of habituation.

Even though Pontanus saw that fear was not appropriate to satire, other scholars have at times noted fear's usefulness in the form of presenting warning examples. Robortello mentioned (by quoting Cicero) that inveterate customs were difficult to change except by scaring people with frightening examples drawn by the satirists (1970, p. 505). In addition to producing fear, satire and tragedy shared other similarities as well. When Aristotle asserted that laughter was essential to comedy, he observed that "the laughter-inducing element is part of the contemptible element and consists of a blunder or silliness not causing distress or disaster" (*Poetics* 1449a; trans. J. H. Meter). Meter argued that when granting comedy a laughter-provoking element that did not cause pain or disaster, Aristotle in fact "effectively disassociated the comical element from the subject matter of satire and tragedy" (1984, p. 109). Thus, satire and tragedy were close in sharing painful subject matter.

Meter also noted that Heinsius, when discussing comedy, was very critical of everything arousing laughter and considered evoking laughter to be reprehensible, unworthy of a wise man and something that appealed to the lower classes.[25] Heinsius objected to laughter from a Platonic–Stoic point of view, whereby laughter was regarded as an expression of uncontrolled emotion: "Of all the emotions laughter is the most intolerable because it signifies a mentality which does not flourish by the prescript of reason but by that of the senses" (1643, p. 17; trans. Meter 1984, p. 109). Laughter was also least subject to moderation. However, Meter interpreted these ideas to mean that Heinsius did not reject laughter as such but only objected to immoderate and unbridled laughter, preferring refined humour. Nevertheless, when Heinsius later came to discuss satirical laughter, he seems to have changed his view of laughter's usefulness and value considerably. Laughter was now harnessed to serve moral correction and purification, and the whole satirical catharsis lay to a great extent in laughter, which was not merely a secondary effect.

To dwell briefly on differences between the genres, satire differed from comedy in being a special mixture of amusement and the two negative emotions, hatred and indignation. This feature was related to the differences between comical and satirical objects: comedy censured hunchbacks and fools, but satire targeted morally bad criminals who posed a threat to society (Taylor 1988, p. 325).[26] Satire and comedy differed in the sense that physical ugliness was not a sufficient source of satirical laughter as it was in comedy, but moral deficiency and actual vice – human cruelty, immoral excesses, fanaticism and other serious social vices and concerns – were also required. This was also realised in the proper targets of satire listed in Renaissance poetics. As typical satirical targets, Robortello named ambitious, greedy, ungrateful, extravagant, perjured, rapacious, adulterous, smooth-tongued, loquacious, stupid, affectionate, tasteless, irreligious, treasonable, lazy and parasitic human beings

(1970, p. 501). In Pontanus's poetics these conventional types recurred: Satire ridiculed and censured people who were idle, parasitic, deformed, loquacious, ungrateful, libidinous, drunken and greedy; he also named usurers, assassins, thieves and adulterers (1594, p. 171). Although both galleries of satirical objects included many merely ridiculous character types, satirical targets often bore serious moral defects and invited the audience to deliberate seriously about morals, whereas in comedy, real vices were absent and the audience was distanced from moral implications (Taylor 1988, p. 325). The moral deficiency required of the satirical target also meant that satirical laughter was not only as pleasurable and amusing as the laughter evoked by comedy, but also more painful. The negative features induced stronger negative emotions and reactions to vices in the audience.

What then can we conclude from these discussions of satirical catharsis? First, we should note that satirical purging was directed to human vices and wrong human actions. The undesirable content that was thereby eliminated was the excess or extremes of vice and passion. Christoph Deupmann has recently argued that satirical catharsis differed significantly from tragic catharsis in the sense that harmful emotions were counteracted by their opposite and beneficial emotions, whereas in tragedy the same emotions that were produced in the audience were also the objects of purification (2002, p. 110). But the theory of satirical catharsis held by Heinsius and his followers was in fact more complex and included various ways of purification, since satires differed from each other. Some were intended to moderate the excess of passions and vices, whereas others were more reluctant to accept any passions and in the Stoic manner regarded all passions as vices. By referring to modern studies we can also claim that compared with the comic purgation the object of the satirical purifying process is different, since comic laughter expels such bad feelings as anxiety, envy, fear, melancholy, sexual aggression or hostility, but not truly serious vices.[27]

The process of satiric catharsis may also be compared with its tragic equivalent, where the emotions of fear and pity were both produced by the tragedy and then therapeutically relieved and purged by watching the same play. But when tragedy imitated action and a man was deemed happy or unhappy with respect to what he did or suffered, satire worked through warning examples, character imitation and blame according to a character's personal qualities.[28] The purified mind in question belonged to the satirical target, but also the author and his audience were considered to be patients needing to be restored to moral health. Their disturbing emotions were altered when laughter diminished their indignation and hatreds, and the warning examples deterred them from vicious actions. There were thus at least two processes taking place: the purging from vices and the purging from hatred and indignation, the feelings of satire proper. It is worth noting that the satirical emotions were very strong, intensive and, apart from laughter, negative, not pleasurable, similar to a bitter pill offered by a medical doctor.

The word "purging" was also related to different phases of the satirical experience. Heinsius explicitly called the purging of the human mind (1) the purpose (*finis*) of satire, but it can also be understood as (2) the end result of the process, which takes place in the audience after its members have followed the satiric representation of the negative examples and have learned to avoid vices. On the other hand, purgation was also used in (3) the therapeutic process, which the audience undergoes in the satirical experience.[29] This process can modify all vices and emotions considered harmful or only their excesses and the most detrimental passions. The process can be started by different means. Therefore, the purgation has also been related to (4) the different cathartic methods used by the satirists. As we have seen, purging acquired different forms according to the three different philosophical schools and their ethical models. According to Heinsius and Volpi, Horace's satires especially used the cathartic method proper and were responded to with *animorum expiatio*. This did not mean merely alteration of the emotions but also the gaining of cognition.

In practice, satires evoked very different emotions. For example, in Heinsius's time Calvinist preachers took a strict stand against poetry (and theatre in particular) in the Netherlands as well as in England, France and Switzerland (Meter 1984, pp. 36–7). Satire was even more difficult to take than other forms of poetry because it described vices and used dirty words. The contemporary religious atmosphere was one big reason for writers like Heinsius to provide a moral justification of the art of satire and other genres. Obscene passages and words that elsewhere aroused indignation towards the speaker were justified as being useful in censuring the sinful target and as a means of moral instruction. Rigault (1684) mentioned that anatomical terms, words pointing to intimate body parts and their functions (such as the vulva or urinary bladder) were essential to satirical criticism and its parrhesia. Satirists had a special licence to use words related to defecation, urination and the genitals; these were part of the genre's purifying equipment. Not all authors of poetics agreed, however. For example, Giovanni Antonio Viperano (1535–1610), a Sicilian historian and humanist, wrote in his *De poetica libri tres* (1579) that "the satiric poet ought especially to avoid all filthy subjects and words, lest attempting to purge minds of dirt, he contaminate them with even fouler blemishes" (1987, p. 141; trans. Philip Rollinson). He advised that satire should maintain purity and elegance in diction.[30] Likewise, Pontanus cautioned that "satirical jokes and wit should do without thematic and verbal obscenity; instead they should censure crimes and desires so that while purging the minds of the guilty, they would not at the same time induce ugliness of manners into sincere and innocent minds" (1594, p. 172).

Therapy as punishment

Even though the satirists often had at least the pretext of healing, considering the actual practice it would be misleading to take this as the whole truth. Mary Claire Randolph has noted that the Renaissance satirist's most common guise was that of the barber-surgeon, who sought to cure malignant swellings and contagious diseases, which represented vice and folly. But even when the satirist's ink was thought to cure, at the same time it bit like acid, salt or wormwood, and the satirist's pen often turned into a cauterizing scalpel or a whip, which inflicted deep scars on the victim's skin (Randolph 1941, p. 145). The images of anatomical dissection and purging with laxatives and other drugs were used in characterising satire as well (pp. 147–8). Satirical treatment was thought to be painful but beneficial; it was never used merely to ease the pain.

Ancient authors had long ago recognised the punitive aspect of wise words. Plato declared in his *Gorgias* (477–9) that the sick person was better off treated than not, although punishing of the soul and relieving its sickness often aroused unpleasant feelings (cf. Lloyd 2003, p. 143). In satires the pain was caused by the biting truth, represented in the images of medical treatment and the harsh words of the doctor who crudely revealed the patient's true physical condition. The verb of wounding and the act of scraping the diseased skin (*radere*) with a surgical knife in order to purify the putrefying flesh were repeatedly applied in characterising the genre in Roman satire (cf. Persius 1.107; 5.15). A scholiast called attention to the technical sense of the verb by saying that the satirist attacked and corrected immoral habits by punishing those who indulged in them, precisely as doctors healed a wound that had begun to fester.[31] The Roman satirists also aggressively attacked inner weaknesses, for instance, by pulling old biases out of his patient's lungs and commanding him to learn, *disce* (Persius 5.92). As internal organs, the lungs were close to the soul. The same function was at times performed by other internal organs as well, such as the liver (Persius 5.129, *intus et in iecore aegro*). Lust especially was thought to be situated in the liver (Bramble 1974, p. 90). Thus, the ailing body may literally mean the ailing soul. Landino remarked that the word *praecordia* (breast, diaphragm) used by Horace in his satire (1.4.89) equalled the mind and the soul (1486, *ad loc.*).[32] The harshness of the treatment included vituperations and reproofs against vices and the stacks of warnings addressed to the patient in order to make him shudder. The satirists insisted that the treatment had to be accepted, since it was better to feel some distress than to live an uncorrected life or to escape from unpleasant truths.

In Randolph's view, the background of satire was in primitive magical curses from which literary satires inherited a lethal element and the primitive notion of destroying or harming the human body for revenge. Medical analogy was adopted in a punishing function, too, since medical treatment, drastic remedies, cautery and surgery, whose intent was blasting and destroying the victim's body without sanative purposes, could at worst be merely destructive.[33] Giovanni Gioviano Pontano (1429–1503) described in his *De sermone* (1499), a book on verbal humour and wit, scurrility and malicious scorn as words that "not only bite but also burn and cause pustules and cancers", thus far from the image of healing (1954, III, Caput XIII; cf. Bauer 1986, p. 300). Thomas G. Benedek has argued that diseases and their treatment acquired a punitive role, especially in Renaissance Christian culture, which developed an emphasis on personal guilt. In his view, during the Renaissance medical images were directed at political enemies and the wealthy more often than before (1992, pp. 373–4). Especially in Renaissance and Reformation polemics, satirists gave up their role as healers and acted like sadistic quacks; rather than promoting good health, their objective seemed to be the enjoyment of causing maximal pain with their drugs and instruments. Sadistic doctors no longer cared whether the punishment was justified and suited the patient's lifestyle; on the contrary, they seemed to think that no pain was too much for their victims. Thus, the satirists themselves were in danger of turning into negative characters who represented the overall corruption of a society in which no authority was reliable or just, and no clear order assured the separation between the healthy and the sick.

Nicodemus Frischlin is an interesting case in point. Frischlin was a fiery and bitter satirist who also published commentaries on classical authors (Aristophanes, Callimachus, Horace) and, in 1582, a paraphrase of Persius. Horace's and Persius' styles and phrases strongly affected Frischlin's satires written against a convert, the Catholic Jacob Rabus, even to the extent that he adopted whole passages nearly unaltered from the Roman authors for his own polemics. Among Frischlin's eight satires against Rabus (*Satyrae octo adversus Iacobum Rabum*, c. 1567–68), the second and the third in particular were composed by adopting specific medical phrases from Persius' poems. In the manner of his Roman predecessors, Frischlin dreamed of removing the victim's glossy skin (*pellem qua Rabus amictus* / [...] *detrahere ut possim*) and revealing his shameful and stupid inside (*intus turpis & excors*); these images were now more threatening and aggressive in tone. Frischlin also pulled foolishness out of the patient's lungs (*nugas tibi de pulmone revellam*) and medicated Rabus's stupid ears (*stupidas mordaci radere vero / auriculas*). Likewise, Persius had rinsed his listener's ears with vinegar, then poured a hot potent drug into the ear, thereby causing it to steam.[34] According to Murmellius's commentary on Persius, the phrase *vaporata aure* was a metaphorical expression primarily used for piping hot flesh taken from the oven (1516, xv^{r}). Since the satirist's patients were suffering from fatal diseases, the medicine had to be like mild acid – undiluted and irritating, with no pleasurable honey coating it. By purifying and steaming the ear canal, the satirist ensured that an easy passage was opened for the Stoic Cleanthes' seed or fruit, as Persius put it (5.63–4).

Persius compared philosophical teaching with ear-cleansing and preparing the way to true knowledge, but Frischlin's therapeutic activities were punishing and not expected to improve the patient's condition. Frischlin asked, why waste effort healing Rabus's intestines when such a patient was made deaf by the Papists' continuous quarrels and unable to hear the satirist's healthy precepts? His skin was completely hardened by his sins and thus prevented the satirist's medicating words from penetrating the inner corners of his sick soul. Frischlin declared that he had abandoned all hope of the victim's sanity (*de Rabi pene salute iam desperatum*) – an expression that contained an obscene pun on Rabus's male member and suggested a potential infection resulting from a venereal disease. The sense of ironic desperation was also reflected in the grammar. In describing his attempts to cure the patient (using verbs like "try to", "attempt to"), Frischlin inflected the therapeutic expressions, writing in the subjunctive form as if expressing an unreal or incurable case. Through this means the satirist stressed the uselessness of his healing efforts.

Frischlin's second satire included a talk given by Gluttony describing the luxurious dishes consumed by Rabus, who despised simple, virtuous nourishment. The poem concluded with a typical death scene of a sick glutton, which once again echoed Persius' fifth satire (5.58–61), but added an image of a worm that represented an unknown evil within: "But when a stony gout (*chiragra*) has smashed your trembling joints / and you have turned painfully grey / and a worm has gradually gnawed its way through your liver, / then you repent of having lived so fatly and having spent your years / in the middle of the sea of crimes" (1607, *sat.* 2). The image of a worm was probably used here because worms were associated with corpses and putrefaction; the image had also been used in Christian polemics.

In the third satire, describing how Rabus began to fall ill, Frischlin's diagnosis was based entirely on terms found in Persius' third satire (3.98–103): the body grew weaker, the limbs trembled with pain, sulphurous belches escaped from the patient's throat and he was short of breath. The characteristic sick paleness was also mentioned as well as his chattering teeth, which the lips had disclosed. Rabus's head was swollen and soaked with drunkenness to the point that his mind was completely darkened. The pessimistic conclusion was that Rabus was firmer in body than in the soul.

Other Renaissance polemics used violent therapy as well. Antonius Codrus Urceus (1446–1500) was a professor and humanist who taught for several years in Bologna. In his second verse satire (1506), written against ignorance, he presented a cure against folly, which became visible, for example, in the symptoms of lethargy and blindness. The cure aimed to correct the patient's lifestyle and contained instruction (*regimen vitae*) for moderation and diet management and also suggested various purgative therapies. Urceus saw that ignorance was based on immoderate living and on the imbalance of the body humours.

A famous humanist satire entitled *Epistolae obscurorum virorum* (1515–17) also described how the obscure scholastics suffered from indigestion, great intumescences in the lower body and other disturbances of the intestines that reflected their mental and moral confusion (Kivistö 2002, pp. 190–216). As an antidote, they were ordered to follow moderation in all activities and observe certain dietary regulations. Purgation therapy, as if to parody the satirical purifying method, was also used: Mammotrectus Buntemantellus, for example, who was suffering from love-sickness was force-fed a cleansing against his will, which resulted in five Gargantuan s(h)ittings that kept him up all night long.

These popular letters were soon imitated in the anonymous *Eccius dedolatus* ("Eck the sculpted") of 1520, a satirical play composed in the Aristophanic tradition to deride and attack Johann Eck (Johann Maier, 1486–1543), a theologian from Ingolstadt. Eck was known as one of Luther's most notorious opponents, who had protested Luther's ninety-five theses and in 1517 compiled a complaint called *Obelisks*, to which Luther had responded the next year with his rebuttal entitled *Asterisks*. Eck had also demanded that Luther's books be confiscated and burned in 1520; thus, he came to be represented as an archconservative by the Reformation-minded humanist satirists.[35]

The main setting of the play was the Ingolstadt home of Eckius. It opened with his parodical lamentations, bemoaning his agony and suffering from a consuming fever represented very much in the manner of Lucian's mock-tragedy *Tragodopodagra*.[36] Eckius groaned about the "cruel curse" of torturing fire that inflamed his viscera, affected his joints and flowed forth from his innermost being. His boy servant philosophised and reminded him – in the manner of Horace's impertinent slave Damasippus – that had Eckius been satisfied with water, he would not be suffering so painfully. Then, after having once again tried an unsuccessful cure with wine and Saxon beer, having found no relief through the help of friends – represented as if by a chorus in the play – and having rejected several unsuitable doctors as potentially dangerous, Eckius sent for an expert surgeon recommended by his friends, a group of Leipzig theologians, to heal him.

The "expert" arrived riding a smelly goat and accompanied by the witch and sorceress, Canidia, who is also known from Horace's epodes and satires. The trip by air (1971, p. 49; 1931, pp. 79–80) included an overtly scatological passage in which Eckius's friend Johannes Rubeus, travelling on the same goat, was forced to relieve his bowels (the day before he had avidly consumed fresh-brewed beer). The surgeon's outward appearance hardly reassured Eckius: he was wearing silver rings instead of gold, a sign of his inferiority to physicians who treated with conventional medicine. Surgery was a treatment of last resort; likewise, surgeons were often derided as an exceptionally brutal group who enjoyed the sadistic pleasures of dissecting (Wagner 1993, p. 212). And indeed, when asked about his healing methods, the surgeon boasted of having cured a myriad of earlier patients so thoroughly by his fire, iron, wheel and rope that they never fell sick again. Violence was involved: "Anything that was irremediable I cut away: I lopped off the tongue of some, gouged out the eyes of others, and suppressed the pruritus of some with switches" (1971, p. 51, trans. Thomas W. Best; 1931, p. 81).

What followed was a conventional diagnostic inspection: examination of the patient's pulse, which was found to be slow and weak, and observation of the colour, odour and consistency of his urine, which appeared bad-smelling, extremely meagre and pale. In the expert's eyes these characteristics indicated necrosis, burning fever, incipient delirium, excess of black bile and possibly insanity, phrenitis, fatuity and frenzy. In the surgeon's concluding words, death was imminent. Further pathological symptoms observed by the surgeon echoed the imagery of Roman verse satire; the disease had put down deep roots and was lurking under the skin, down in the viscera (1971, p. 53; 1931, p. 83, *morbus enim altius radices egit; omnis vis mali in praecordiis et sub cute latet*). The bad condition ensued from a number of different sins, including intoxication, lust, anger, envy and craving for fame, which a confessor detected in Eckius before the actual treatment began (1971, pp. 54–7; 1931, pp. 84–5). Fault was also found with the patient's theological principles, which were preoccupied with ceremonies, Scotus's subtleties and Thomas's solidities (1971, pp. 58–9; 1931, pp. 87–8).

The culmination of the satire was Eckius's violent therapy (1971, pp. 64–70; 1931, pp. 91–6), which skipped over the milder treatments of dietary regulations and medication and concentrated on surgical action. First, the patient's rough edges and "angles" (a pun on Eck's name) were soundly beaten and softened by seven strong men. Then the patient was tied to his bed, his head was shaved and sophisms, syllogisms, propositions, corollaries and other scholastic trifles hiding there were expelled. The theologian's ears were cleansed, the black and forked tongue cut off and a gigantic canine tooth pulled out. The surgeon repeated diagnostic words from Roman satire, frequently stressing that the entire defect or ulceration was hiding inside and under the skin (*intus et sub cute lateat*); therefore, the patient had to be skinned like Marsyas who was flayed alive. Before the operation he was offered a soporific draught to ease the pain, which also caused vomiting and purged his belly of the poorly digested commentaries on the logical and physical works of Aristotle, which Eck had himself written; the excrement also included some coins from the collected indulgences. The act of removing the skin, familiar as a metaphor from Roman satire, was here carried out literally. The pestilential ulcers that were burned or cut off from his open breast included arrogance, sycophancy, vainglory, slander, dissolution, deceit, hypocrisy and similar sins. After all this beating, purging, cutting and other violently therapeutic operations, the surgeon finally turned his knife against the worst ulcer of all and emasculated the patient (1971, p. 70; 1931, p. 96). Similar violent initiations of new students, the so-called *depositio beani*, took place at German universities, as will be noted later. The play turned out to be a comedy, since Eckius was absolved from his sins and cured.

Barbara Könneker (1991, pp. 161–2) has noted that similar treatments were to be found in the *Narrenschneiden* familiar from Hans

Sachs's Shrovetide plays, in the sick patients of Thomas Murner's *Narrenbeschwörung* and other contemporary *Narrenliteratur.* Frischlin's famous philological comedy *Priscianus vapulans* (1585) also contained doctors and different forms of linguistic purification. *Eccius dedolatus* also had its imitators. Eduard Böcking (1860) edited two short, anonymous dialogues, *Decoctio* and *Eckius monachus*, written shortly after *Eccius dedolatus* and having the same central figure. Böcking suggested in his preface to *Eccius dedolatus* that the texts were written by a medical doctor, since they included detailed medical knowledge. But they could just as well have been simple rewritings of the earlier satirical therapies. In *Decoctio* the two patients were Eck and a certain Leus, who had attacked Erasmus. Both suffered from pallor caused by too much cumin (implying pretence of learning)[37] and Huttenian fever (a form of insanity). At first, they were deemed incurable in their insanity, but Podalyrius, the son of Aesculapius was called for. He prepared a strong medicinal draft in which Eck and Leus were forced to bathe naked. At that point the force of the medicine made strange creatures rush out of their ears, while their departing folly released foul odours, until they were finally pronounced purged and cured through having suffered maximal pain. That they had recovered sanity and been restored to their senses was noted in the praises they now sang of Luther and Erasmus.

As the previous pages have shown, purity of mind and composure of moral health could be achieved either by means of punitive correction, in which the physician-satirist compelled the patient to go through painful treatment, or by more therapeutic means, in which healthy precepts and instructive words were offered by the philosopher-satirist. Likewise, the method of purgation had both the high Aristotelian purpose of satire as pronounced in poetics, and also concrete scatological sessions in the satires themselves through which the patient-victims were to be "cured", that is, improved. The acts of forced vomiting and violence described above had their predecessors in Roman verse satire, but also in such Menippean works as Lucian's *Lexiphanes* and Martianus Capella's *De nuptiis Philologiae et Mercurii* (cf. Relihan 1993, pp. 144–5). In Lucian's dialogue (18–21), a physician called Sopolis purges a linguistic pedant by giving him medicine made for an insane person and by forcing him to throw up his high-sounding vocabulary. In Martianus Capella's satire Philology drinks an emetic, which purges her of great heaps of literature and learning (2.135–9). And later an old woman – Grammar – acts like a skilled physician and by using a pruning knife and other sharp medicines heals children of bucolic ignorance and solecisms (3.223–6).

In the following pages, I will deal with texts in which especially the impact of Lucian's satirical dialogues becomes notable, his influence being evident, for example, in Ulrich von Hutten's (1488–1523) dialogues on fever, *Febris I–II*, or in the influential *Apologia seu Podagrae laus* (1522), which was probably the earliest Renaissance gout eulogy and written by the Nuremberg humanist Willibald Pirckheimer (1470–1530); these works were written in the aftermath of Lucian's *Podagra*.

3
Painfully Happy: Satirical Disease Eulogies and the Good Life

According to Johannes Britannicus, one of the most prominent vices censured in satire – luxury – owed its name to twisted body parts, which were distorted from their normal positions, just as luxurious habits were dissolute and turned from their regular course.[1] Satires described various pathological symptoms – paleness, wounds, stomach pains, excess bile, fever and gout – which bespoke questionable living habits and were said to be the well-deserved consequences. Gout especially was the subject of several satirical texts in the early modern period, because it was thought to result from self-indulgent, luxurious living and hence, was called a rich man's malady (cf. Juvenal 13.96, *locupletem podagram*), since it usually affected wealthy and highly esteemed men.

However, analogies of diseases and physical infirmities have not always been drawn with mental or moral weakness nor has disease always been used as a vehicle for condemning an immoral target. In this chapter I examine diseased bodies that, instead of simply indicating a corrupted condition or representing vices, were more ambiguous and also paradoxically praised as being connected with virtue. Balde characterised gout in his *Solatium podagricorum seu lusus satyricus* (1661, poem 53) in ambivalent terms: "Gout is clearly a disease in which contrasts meet: it is friendly fury, the sweet ignorance of old age, militant peacefulness, flame that does no damage, miserable marriage, tame syphilis, funeral comedy, fables acted out wearing socks but without ordinary speech, ridiculous pain [...]". Balde pointed out that the sensations aroused by gout were not merely an annoyance in people's lives. He called gout a paradox granted by the gods, which blessed a man by leaving him without the joys of living (poem 35). His contemporary satirists shared his view and discussed gout in positive terms, either on grounds that it was a just punishment for sins or because it could actively work as a painful but beneficial healer. In the latter function, diseases and physical weaknesses were regarded as positive qualities, which concealed true beauty, moral health and virtue and which advanced the achievement of spiritual strength and the good life.

In the following sections I will explain the logic behind such claims. Since the genre of disease encomium drew upon both rhetoric and philosophy, I will examine first the rhetorical background of these discussions and then focus in more detail on certain specific diseases and praises of them from the playfully philosophical point of view.

Epideictic rhetoric and paradoxical praises of disease

Paradoxical praises of disease were often written by medical doctors who had professional interests in the disease or who had composed a speech for a graduation ceremony, the opening of the academic year or some other university occasion (Siraisi 2004, p. 193). These orations ranged from earnest medical readings to playful Lucianic imitations, the most common topic being praise of medicine in general. One important argument in such speeches was that medicine improved the welfare of the mind and the morals. In his *Medicinae encomium* (1559), Girolamo Cardano (1501–76) praised the utility, beauty and nobility of medicine and stated that no one would call into question the divinity of Christ; yet Christ performed nothing more than medicine, healing patients, albeit in a divine way. In Cardano's view, the benefits of medicine also included the wealth acquired in the profession; expulsion of superstitious causes of illnesses, such as demons; restoring men to life and its pleasures; and the longevity of doctors (Hippocrates lived for one hundred years; Avenzoar for nearly one hundred and thirty). Owing to their verbal presentation, the structure of such eulogies was often loose, circling around the main theme and assembling familiar historical examples and recognisable commonplaces to support and illustrate the point the author wished to make.

These speeches had their immediate context in epideictic oratory and its two sub-genres, praise and blame. Serious praises usually eulogised great men, virtues, beautiful cities or highly esteemed fields of knowledge; their subject was something that was seen as good and noble (Lausberg 1998, §243). Epideictic oratory asked the audience to make judgements of good and bad and usually to share the evaluations it represented. Thus, epideictic oratory could serve as an instrument to achieve of moral ends and, in the manner of satire, supply examples of good and bad conduct while praising virtues and blaming vices. Plato memorably said that hymns to the gods and praises of famous men were useful in the best possible republic, since they produced emotions that were not perturbed or hedonistic but profitable, such as hunger for fame. Such praises strengthened the state by stimulating desire for emulating virtue and making vice seem unattractive. Although the goods of nature – family, beauty, riches and other favours of fortune – were also extolled, the true objects of praise were noble deeds and virtue achieved by a person's conduct. Praise was the verbal expression of a man's good qualities.

By contrast, paradoxical encomia challenged orthodox opinions and asserted the relativity of all value judgements. Instead of defending the obvious, paradoxical praises eulogised things that were commonly regarded as vile, harmful or indefensible. These objects could include anything that was small (insects, vermin and small animals), trivial (nuts, vegetables and pot-herbs), deformed (dwarfs, ugly faces), immoral (moral evils, promiscuity, drunkenness) or difficult to bear (diseases, imprisonment, suicide, injustice, Nero). Also larger mammals, flowers and abstract concepts such as nothingness, something or darkness were frequently treated. Incongruence that was formed between the epideictic mode and the unexpected object of praise created surprise and humour.[2]

By presenting vile things in a favourable light, paradoxical encomia amused and provoked the audience's thinking. In their defence of something ugly or shameful, paradoxical speeches were called *turpe genus* (in *Rhetorica ad Herennium*), which disturbed the audience's sense of decorum, virtue and even justice. Another generic name used in this connection was *admirabile* (*figura paradoxos id est admirabilis,* by Fortunatus), since now the audience felt its general sense of value and truth to be challenged (Lausberg 1998, §64.3). By focusing on a low or depraved subject, paradoxical encomia drew attention to certain conventional limits of the audience's thinking and their opinions of the traditional values of things and standards by which these values were established.[3] The rejection of the opinion of the multitude was an argument that was repeatedly expressed and shared by philosophers and paradoxical authors as well.

As for the representational conventions of the genre, Erasmus had announced his inspirers and sources at the beginning of his *Moria*; thereafter, it became customary to express consciousness of the famous literary parentage and thereby to make acceptable one's own interest in such frivolous literary activity (Tomarken 1990, p. 49). Disease eulogies like Johannes Carnarius's (Jan de Vleeschouwer, 1527–62) *De podagrae laudibus oratio* (1553) alluded to standard classical authorities, such as Lucian, Synesius, Favorinus' encomium of quartan fever and Cicero's praises of old age, pain and death (1619, p. 220).[4] Paradoxical praises reused arguments and commonplaces from earlier works, and they were conventionally structured. Often they mined their mythological and historical examples, proverbs and source references from different fields, but preferred quoting highly esteemed authors and philosophers like Aristotle, Cicero and Seneca. For instance, physical weakness was praised by appealing to the example of Plato who, according to some legends, lived in an unhealthy region of Athens for the purpose of strengthening his mind; Plato believed that a stronger body weakened the strength of the mind. In his *Medicinae encomium*, Cardano objected to this idea and argued that such stories were told merely for the sake of rhetoric and paradoxes. He assumed that Plato simply wanted to live in peaceful isolation in order to concentrate on his philosophy.

Paradoxical disease eulogies aspired to offer an antidote to patients' sorrows. The authors argued that patients should replace grief and suffering with reasoning and happiness, since disease or disability was not a real cause of evil but, on closer examination, a blessing in disguise. The arguments in favour of disease were usually based on the same qualities and virtues that were found in the praises of great men and beautiful cities – moral value, honour, nobility, usefulness and beauty (Lausberg 1998, §247; Quintilian, *Institutio oratoria* 3.7.27). Thus, the eulogies minimised the unattractive side or harmful effects of diseases on human beings. Authors spoke of the utility of diseases in forming individual moral character which, when developed, was beneficial to the whole of society. In mapping the virtuous effects of diseases, paradoxical praises shared the edifying purpose with serious panegyrics, but their general tone was always playful, and they parodically employed examples from philosophical discussions, such as the pleasure of scratching. The intention was not merely to ridicule these serious and great thoughts, but also to offer philosophical medicine in a humorous form.

The philosophical background was clearly discernible in the paradox form. Paradox meant a statement that ran contrary to general opinion (Balde 1658b, p. 44: *paradoxum, a communi sensu alienum*). *Podagraegraphia*, for example, claimed that ordinary people often made mistakes in their perceptions, believing a mountain to be green or an underwater stake to be curved if these seemed so; in the same way they were mistaken about the value of disease (p. 230).[5] Paradoxical encomia (and satire) shared with philosophy the emphasis on the importance of seeing the true values of things beneath their exteriors, and stressed the superiority of the internal and permanent as opposed to the external and accidental. Writers of paradoxes thus defended disease against the audience's habitual expectations, claiming that these general beliefs conflicted with the truth about virtue and happiness. Thereby, the satirists argued that the harmfulness of disease was a mere conventional judgement, based on false opinions and deceptive appearances.

Thus, in satirical disease eulogies philosophical arguments for the good life and rhetorical methods in displaying these arguments interestingly coincided, so that both these traditions – philosophy and rhetoric, which have often been seen as antagonistic in the sense of concentrating on content and form, respectively – constituted a fruitful joint background to the texts discussed here. The issue proposed by rhetoric that virtue was the only true grounds for praise was connected with ethics and philosophical questions about the difference between true and merely ornamental sources of happiness, such as health, riches, power or pleasures. In both discourses internal qualities and virtues were valued as far more important than the gifts of fortune. Illness was a downfall that stripped the patient of many ornamental goods, but at the same time showed him what was truly valuable in his life.

Herewith I will elucidate a handful of texts and arguments that have been presented in favour of three common diseases in the early modern age, namely, fever, gout and the itch. When distinguishing four degrees of defensibility in praises, Menander Rhetor argued that moral evils tolerated no playfulness, whereas lighter issues that did not deserve praise (like poverty or dogs) could be playfully treated (Lausberg 1998, §241).[6] Thus, not even paradoxical encomia usually sought justification for lethal diseases, but praised illnesses that were not contagious – Erasmus, for example, thanked kidney stones for this (1619, p. 202) – and were not fatal to the patient, although they were often chronic and annoying.[7] Sensory disabilities were treated in ancient philosophy, and these arguments were often employed in learned praises as well; sensory defects will be studied in Chapter 4. Venereal diseases were believed to result from intemperate living, but they were praised far less frequently and did not offer material for philosophical consideration; therefore, they will be excluded from this reading.[8] By analysing selected early modern texts, I intend to show how paradoxical encomia put abstract values in concrete form, how these encomia were structured and how they reflected philosophical discussions of virtues and the good life. By arguing that diseases improved individual morality, these eulogies opened up new, albeit playful possibilities for approaching the good life and perhaps helped to put things in a slightly different light.

Fever as a moral disease

Chrysippus of Soli had compared the diseased soul to the feverish body, in which fevers and chills occurred irregularly and at random. Similarly, the diseased soul was attacked by the irrational and unpredictable outbreaks of affections comparable to quartan fever, which did not occur daily but came at intervals (Tieleman 2003, pp. 106–7, 155). In his *De remediis utriusque fortunae* (1354–66), Petrarch claimed that the fevers of the soul were much more dangerous than those of the body (I.4). The authors who praised physical fever often based their paradoxical arguments on such philosophical and medical views of the disease's nature. Favorinus, a Greek rhetorician from the first century, is known as the first author to eulogise fever, perhaps to sharpen his oratorical skills, and he was regularly mentioned by name in Renaissance disease panegyrics. Favorinus' eulogy has not been preserved for us to read, but Aulus Gellius (*Noctes Atticae* 17.12) tells us that Favorinus alluded to Plato who had said that after having recovered from quartan fever, he afterwards enjoyed more constant health. This was a typical argument in fever eulogies: its attacks made the patient stronger than he was before the disease. Fever belonged to the themes used in declamations, and according to Epictetus, if any hardship like fever befell the philosopher Agrippinus, he composed a eulogy upon it (Epictetus, frg. 21; quoted in Billerbeck and Zubler 2000, p. 14).

Although today we know that malaria is transmitted by mosquitoes, in Hippocratic medicine mosquito bites were not considered the cause of fever; instead its reasons were found in the imbalance of the bodily humours (Sallares 2002, pp. 49–50). For the same reason fever was a potentially fruitful disease for moral critics, because the concept of imbalance was related to vices and living habits; therefore, fever too could be interpreted as a moral disease caused by a sinful lifestyle rather than by insects. Renaissance medicine still acknowledged the role of humours in generating fevers. Laurent Joubert (1529–82), a French humanist and medical doctor from Montpellier, argued in his treatise *De quartanae febris generatione* (1567) that quartan fever was produced by melancholic fluid. A moderate diet was crucial in preventing quartan fever, because lavish meals, salted meat, sausages and fresh milk gave rise to thick and crude humours in the body (Caput V). Immoderate use of vinegar, which young girls liked to pour on lettuce and bread, was mentioned as another cause of quartan fever (Caput VII). Joubert's treatise also contained other traditional ideas, for example, about the impact of the season on fevers. Juvenal had already voiced the old belief that severe diseases occurred in the deadly season of autumn (4.57). When the healthier season of the winter months began, people hoped for better times and quartan fevers, which were rarely fatal. Here quartan fever was a sign of a good turn in life. But it was also noted that the fever was often latent for a long time, secretly hiding in the body and difficult to cure unless diagnosed in the first days of its occurrence (Mancinellus and Badius Ascensius 1515, cxi^{r}).

In discussing literary representations of fever, it is worth noting that in the ancient world, Fever as a personification was not a literary invention but a Roman *numen*, a local, very old patronness goddess in Rome who belonged to a group of hostile divinities. She was invoked by the Romans to stop her from exercising power. She probably personified malaria. She was worshipped in high and thus healthier places and on hills – the Palatine, Esquiline and Quirinal – perhaps because fever and malaria were thought to have their origins in low places; the stagnant waters of the river Tiber especially caused frequent fever epidemics around Rome. The Romans propitiated the goddess by building temples and erecting altars to her. The Quartanae were at times given as the daughters of Febris and Saturn. There were also other divinities associated with malaria and fever, such as Dea Tertiana who was mentioned in inscriptions.[9]

As a literary figure, Fever appeared in ancient literature only once, in Seneca's satire *Apocolocyntosis* (6) in which she accompanied the dead Emperor Claudius into the next world and claimed to know his personal history thoroughly after having lived with him for so many years. She seemed to be familiar with the intimate details of Claudius' life, for which reason the Emperor, wishing to decapitate the outspoken goddess, made gestures for her neck to be severed. But no one paid attention. In his essay "Advice about keeping well" (*Moralia* 129A), Plutarch also mentioned the figure of Fever lurking at the door, thus using the image of a *malum* that was seriously threatening the patient who should have taken care of his health beforehand.[10]

According to Alessandro Perosa (1946, pp. 74–5), Fever was reintroduced into literature as late as 1473 by Angelo Poliziano in his occasional poem composed on the death of a young girl, Albiera degli Albizzi (the poem was first published in 1498). In Poliziano's elegy, Fever represented the forces of evil. At the request of Nemesis, Fever entered the girl's bedroom when night fell and instilled into her veins a poison mixed from flames and icy snow and thus killed her. Fever became an evil and malicious character, who punished her victims unto death. Interestingly, in Cunaeus's *Sardi venales* (1612), Poliziano and fever were again brought together. The narrator in Cunaeus's satire – an account of dream visions and imaginary travels – recalled how Poliziano had participated in a discussion in the Underworld about intellectual decline and the spread of the infection of bad authors and their feverish (*febriculosum*) verses (1620, p. 44). In this connection Poliziano had made a speech about the Abderites (originally the inhabitants of Abdera, who were reproached for being stupid; hence, the term was used for all men of such a kind; it was also the birthplace of Democritus). The Abderites were afflicted with fever, caused by the star Sirius, and after seven days they were delirious. The signs of insanity included stylistic distortion, tragic verses and iambs filling the poets' mouths. The delirium lasted until winter set in and the disease gradually lost its strength. The critique presented here against contemporary poetry nicely combined elements from earlier literary history, with reference to universal sickness (*omnium morbus*), Poliziano's poem on fever and the Juvenalian mention of the healthier winter season. Cunaeus also described the philosophers' grove in the Underworld, where doctors of the sciences perambulated in a learned manner (p. 31). Their faces turned pale from scholarly envy whenever other teachers enjoyed a wider audience; jealousy created a chronic fever in them, understood here as a general term for disease. When a philosopher opened his mouth to give a speech, several corybantic and sesquipedalian words were heard (p. 50). This prompted Menippus to call for a doctor to diagnose such a difficult sickness. The doctor ordered continuous perambulations and vomiting to purge the insanity and destroy the tumour.

The narrative structure of a dream vision and intellectual or divine gatherings, loosely modelled on Seneca's *Apocolocyntosis*, was frequently used in contemporary Menippean satire. Rigault's *Funus parasiticum* opened with a discussion of Lucius the ass in a dream (cf. De Smet 1996, pp. 117–50). Justus Lipsius's *Somnium* (1581) famously described a dream set in ancient Rome, where ancient authors and modern grammarians gathered to discuss the commentaries on classical texts. Cicero, Ovid, Varro and others complained that modern authors mutilated their learning; the Roman elegists' guts were torn out and Martial was completely dismembered. Commentators' glossophilia was a pathological symptom, causing wounds and scars to their textual bodies, and several indicators of modern authors' cultural decadence were framed in the language of medical diagnosis. The suggested cures varied from exile to hellebore according to the seriousness of the injury.[11]

After Poliziano, the figure of Fever was encountered in Ulrich von Hutten's two short satirical dialogues *Febris prima* (1518) and *Febris secunda* (1519).[12] According to Lewis Jillings (1995, p. 1), Hutten was the first to use disease as metaphor in a polemical way. In using the disease image, Hutten attacked those whose activities, in his view, threatened the well-being of German society. He wrote about ulcerous theologians, and he willed gout or the French disease upon his luxuriously living contemporaries. Hutten, who himself suffered from syphilis and wrote about his treatments – and hence, frequently made references to the shortcomings of the medical profession – suggested a causal link between the French disease and the consumption of luxurious foreign foods.

In Hutten's *Febris prima* (printed in Böcking 1860, pp. 29–41), the author not only used personification of an illness, but also placed himself in the dialogue as a character, discussing with Fever who wished to enter the household. Hutten-the-interlocutor told Fever to go elsewhere, to spare him and instead take up residence among the rich and among those who had committed crimes and deserved to be punished. Potential patients included men who had given themselves to the pleasures of the flesh – princes, merchants and the "Fuggers" (Augsburg financiers). However, Fever rejected rich men and wealthy townsfolk, since they were already afflicted by gout and many diseases from over-eating and were surrounded by numerous doctors. Simple folk and labourers were also unsuitable hosts, since their hunger and hard work were not conducive to fevers. By way of attacking religious abuses and luxurious living, Hutten persuaded Fever to find her home in the house of papal legate and cardinal Tommaso de Cajetan. Hutten suggested Cajetan along with corrupted catholic priests and fat monks as proper targets for Fever's attacks; *they* were in need of punishment and moral improvement. Conventional advice about abstinence, exercise, sobriety and hard work were given as the means of repelling the fever. Finally, Fever settled for a German cleric and courtier who had recently returned from a cardinal's court in Rome and there, had learned dissolute living. The cardinal mentioned here, Tommaso de Cajetan, was a Dominican theologian who wrote commentaries to Thomas Aquinas, was appointed cardinal in 1517 and after having drafted a bull against Luther in 1520, became one of Hutten's enemies (Benedek 1992, p. 366, n. 51; Best 1969, pp. 62–3). Hutten's attacks on him continued in the dialogue *Inspicientes* (1520). The title of the dialogue refers to Lucian's *Contemplantes* and the term *episkopoi* in general (cf. Robinson 1979, p. 113), but it also includes the diagnostic term familiar from Persius' and Seneca's moral writings. In the dialogue *Vadiscus* (1520), Hutten also attacked Roman Catholics: even if their heads could be preserved, he wrote, the severe disease inside had to be eradicated by a smart doctor using severe pain.

In *Febris secunda* (printed in Böcking 1860, pp. 103–44), Fever returned to Hutten's door and complained that the courtier's house was so crowded with other maladies such as syphilis and gout that she could not possibly stay there. Hutten and his servant once again tried to persuade her to leave, appealing to their sober lifestyle: they only drank boiled water, they said, ate lentils and practiced a Pythagorean mode of living. The dialogue caricatured the clergy's mistresses, concubines and general corruption and called for the moral renewal of the Church. Marriage was discussed as well. Fever advised Hutten never to marry, since taking a wife would mean the end of his studies. Moreover, with a wife's tender care, the beneficial attacks of Fever would be repelled as well. Here, Fever announces that she extinguishes lust. In *Febris prima*, Fever was already viewed as morally beneficial, since during her earlier six-month-long visit in Hutten's place she had taught him the value of industriousness, piety and patience (p. 33). Now she repeats these claims of her usefulness: she makes the patients industrious, sharpens their wits and controls their passions. By transforming the body, she also created a credible appearance for an intellectual: she generated facial pallor, serious outlook and thinness, all associated with ardent study and the scholarly life. Such visible intelligence also appealed to women, as she well knew. Finally, however, she was forced to admit that Hutten, already being extremely learned, did not need her instructive presence; therefore, she decided to travel to Rome where Catholics were always in need of moral and intellectual improvement.[13]

As Lewis Jillings has also observed (1995, pp. 8–9), in another dialogue, entitled *Bulla vel Bullicida* (1520, printed in Böcking 1860, pp. 309–36), Hutten continued attacking his favourite targets, the vices of papacy and the clerics, describing them as a boil that burst, spewing foul substances. The pun in the title alluded to the bubble as a symbol of vanity, but also to the papal decree (bull) and the medical meaning of the word *bulla* as a boil full of putrid corruption. The interlocutors (including again Hutten himself and Bulla) first discussed the meanings of the word *bulla* (p. 316), until Hutten attacked the boil to cure it. The pestilential filth released from the papal boil when it was beaten included perfidy, treachery, ambition, avarice, hypocrisy, simulation, ostentation, drunkenness, lust and other moral transgressions (p. 331). Finally, the boil was given a funeral.[14]

Bubbles were thus images of vanity and things that do not last, but the word also had its medical meaning – it referred to blisters and vesicles. This double association was also used in an anonymous epigram included in *Iocorum atque seriorum centuriae* and addressed to a *doctor bullatus*, an expert whose professionalism was called into question by this very characterisation (p. 164, CCII). Persius too had described a man lacking conscience in similar physical terms: the man was literally drowned and ceased to send bubbles to the surface (3.32–4). His conscience was so deeply buried, indeed nonexistent, that it sent no signs to the outer world or to the man's own consciousness. In the final stage, breathing, which signalled living and the presence of soul, was lacking, and thus there was no hope for life, life being ironically depicted here as light water bubbles.

Hutten's disease dialogues served his anti-Catholic and anti-Papist polemics and had a political purpose, unlike most other disease eulogies, which were either philosophical and consolatory or merely playful and parodical. In addition to its role in Hutten's dialogues, fever was discussed in Gulielmus Insulanus Menapius's (d. 1561) somewhat longer treatise *Encomium febris quartanae* (1542, printed in Dornau 1619).[15] The fever extolled here was periodic and the mildest of fevers; it recurred every fourth day. Tomarken (1990, pp. 70–1) has noted that the suffering from quartan fever epitomised the ambivalent human condition, for a man cannot do well every day; one day is bad and one day, better. The patient stricken by periodic fever was said to be happier than people in general, because the fever had an interval of two or three good days and only one bad. The fever patient was able to continue moderate living; he could still eat and drink wine as usual. The same reasons were used to defend gout: according to Balde, the intervals between the pain gave sweet pleasure and refreshed the mind, just as seeing a coastline delighted sailors who had for a long time been tossed by storms on the rocky sea surrounded by various monsters (1661, poem 38).

Menapius was a medical student whose work resembled the scientific studies that were frequently written during the Renaissance on different fevers, their symptoms and treatments; these included Daniel Sennert's *De febribus*, Joubert's *De quartana febre*, Lorenzo Bellini's *De febribus* and so on. Menapius's work was similar to these studies in its reliance on ancient medical ideas (Galen, Hippocrates, Celsus) and its more than average attention paid to diagnostics, diet and actual therapy. It also challenged earlier notions of the treatment of excess black bile, which was considered one of the reasons for quartan fever. But although based on medical knowledge, the treatise also contained a eulogising defence of the disease. Menapius declared, for example, that the fever did not cause severe pain or kill, but rather allowed the patient several days of freedom to rest, relax and study. Quartan fever was safe compared to acute fevers that more readily led to death. Psychologically, it was more comforting than other diseases, since there was no reason to be afraid of the final outcome; on the contrary, there were grounds for hope and the prospect of recovery (1619, pp. 183–5).

Comparisons were made with other diseases, which the quartan fever expelled, and the favourable changes that the fever was thought to generate in people's lives were also taken into account. Hutten's Fever had already noted that unlike other diseases, she did not cause unpleasant symptoms such as stench or ulcers or cause deformities or lameness or cramp the joints (cf. Benedek 1992, p. 369). Menapius stressed that quartan fever did not affect the brain or cause delirium, that the appetite remained good and that the patient's physical appearance did not change drastically (p. 186). Wine could be moderately consumed, except for the strong red kind. Thus, fever allowed the patient to carry on his normal life, merely regulating it to some healthy extent. Menapius also discussed contagion and noted that unlike other fevers, which were transmitted by mere touch or an evil eye, the quartan type was not contagious (p. 189). Menapius addressed the issue mainly from the medical viewpoint and did not follow Hutten by introducing fever as a moral punishment. Nevertheless, his treatise was classified among the paradoxical encomia and included both in Dornau's compilation and in the *Admiranda rerum admirabilium encomia*. Its fever had evident moral effects, since it made men both physically and mentally stronger and in this sense improved their health. Menapius stressed that philosophical consolation was unnecessary, because there was no reason to grieve (p. 190).

Medical treatises also recognised several similar advantages of fever. Joubert (1567, Caput XIII) claimed that the body afflicted by fever was expected to achieve a permanent alteration and to become stronger. Moreover, quartan fever usually never seized the same person again. By reference to Galen, Joubert assumed that this was because the evacuations caused by fever were so thorough that there no longer remained any excess fluids – the material for fever to work – in the body. Joubert saw that fever had the power to change men's lifestyles, temperaments and appetites. Thus, fever clearly had cathartic and morally healing effects. Quartan fever did not kill the patient, and it allowed several days of freedom between bouts; thus, it was deemed better than many other diseases. In Joubert's view, rhetoricians, physicians and philosophers had good reasons for their praises of quartan fever.

The characterisations of fever were very different in those epigrams and elegies that lamented the sadness caused by the disease and groaned about the gradual failure of strength in the limbs. The Jesuit poet Johannes Kreihing (1595–1670), for example, imitating Martial and Propertius in his poetry, composed an epigram *De febri sua, et medico* on his deplorable condition and jeered at an indifferent doctor who promised that the poet would not die yet offered no cure (the poem is printed in Mertz 1989, pp. 58–9). This reminds of Petronius' playful saying (*Satyricon* 42) that, after all, a doctor is nothing but consolation for the soul.[16]

Divine gout dwells in wealth and luxury

Gout was another popular topic for ridicule in early modern humorous and satirical texts. Balde, for example, made joking parallels between gout patients' bound feet and his own verses, saying that he had adjusted the poetic form to the topic – the consolation of gout patients' pain – by binding his verses into hexameters which allowed him to take six steps only (1661, question 38). A non-lethal disease that arose from the patients' own vices, gout invited satire, which at times took the form of downright attacks against wealth and luxury, with gout being introduced as a well-deserved punishment for these moral failings. The idea that luxury brought retribution was shared by moral and medical authors alike.

In ancient Hippocratic medicine, gout was regarded as the outcome of the excessive accumulation of bodily humours caused, for example, by sedentary life or sexual excess. The spread of gout to groups of people who had not previously been afflicted was interpreted as a sign of a changed society, one that had abandoned its earlier simplicity. Galen noted that in wicked modern times, even otherwise intact groups, such as eunuchs, women or younger boys, could occasionally contract gout (Porter and Rousseau 1998, pp. 14–15). Seneca argued in his moral epistles (95.20–1) that gout had been a rare disease in the early Republic, but with the spread of luxury and decadence in imperial Rome, gout had become a major problem, even among women, who now were also running the risk of losing their hair. The spread of the disease and the manly appearance of women, including their baldness, were specifically connected with the changed manner of living. For Seneca, the sheer number of cooks was another clear sign of decay. Thus, Johannes Carnarius noted that all individuals who were rich and leisured could fall victim to gout (Tomarken 1990, p. 65). And Balde concurred; even though beardless gout was a rare monster and women were less prone to gout in the feet than to diseases of the head, if they indulged in men's drinking habits they too could be stricken with men's diseases (1661, question 29). As a remedy, medical and moral authors recommended physical exercise and moderation. Spare diet, hard work and abstinence prevented the disease. Although gluttony, drunkenness and other vices were not the exclusive privilege of the wealthy, poor men seldom had gout or other morally-disposed illnesses. Epigram 11.403 in the *Greek Anthology* claimed that gout delighted in draughts of Italian wine and other delicacies that were never found among the poor. In Aristophanes' *Plutus* the personified Poverty claims that the poor enjoy good mental and physical health, whereas the wealthy suffer constantly (cf. Meyer 1915, pp. 3, 13, 39).

An early literary example of this attitude was Lucian's mock-tragedy *Tragodopodagra* in which the characters were a gouty man, the furious goddess Podagra, a chorus of Pains and various medical doctors. In the very first lines (1–29), the gouty man complained of the agony and punishment caused by the disease and compared his lot with the mythological sinners Tantalus and Sisyphus, who had to pay for their wicked deeds with eternal suffering in the Underworld. The tortures caused by gout were explicitly connected with sinful activities. Lucian's gout was a merciless goddess and a dreadful, nearly sadistic ruler who scorned those who wished to avoid her powerful punishment (176–7). Lucian further developed the moral implications of gout when he focused on the disease's effects on people's gait and ability to walk. Lucian's gouty man asked his staff for help supporting his trembling steps, to guide his path aright that he might "place sure feet upon the ground" (55–7; trans. M. D. Macleod). This unsteadiness had moral undertones in the sense of finding the right way of living and of choosing the path of virtue at a crossroads. Firm steps equalled right decisions and a sound mind, whereas the trembling walk typical of gout patients metaphorically illustrated the fundamental uncertainty of all human action, decision-making and moral choices. The sick condition and the unsteady gait can also be readily taken as reminders of inescapable human corporality and mortality.

Other traditional images were also used by Lucian to illustrate the human condition. The metaphors of light and darkness so often applied in drawing distinctions between divine wisdom and imperfect human knowledge were present here as well. The gouty man, forced to stay at home, longed to release his eyes "from deep dark cloud of mist" and go outdoors into the light of the sun (60–1). Entrance into the light was prevented by his feeble body, which did not obey his will. The passage constructed a conventional opposition between body and mind, darkness and light, as moral critics loved to value mind over body and to contrast the animal and divine sides of the human being.

Lucian's text inspired many imitators in early modern literature, where the reason for the illnesses was found in patients' lifestyles. According to various legends, many ancient heroes and demigods had some injury in their feet, for example, due to falling off a horse (Bellerophon), a pin driven through the ankles (Oedipus) or a snake-bite (Philoctetes). These often repeated examples were mined from a similar list given in Lucian's *Tragodopodagra* (250–64), and their purpose was to glorify gout by connecting it to noble men of history. Gout eulogies gave examples of famous ancient Greeks who had suffered from gout, including the classical heroes of Troy (Priam, Ulysses, Achilles) and other mythical figures (Peleus, Bellerophon, Oedipus, Plisthenes, Protesilaus). Willibald Pirckheimer's *Apologia seu podagrae laus* argued that Achilles did not refuse to help the Greeks because of the maiden Briseis, since there never was any Briseis, but because of Gout, who had infected the famous hero and forced him to stay in his tent (2002, §83).

But such lists of royal agonies were also critical of the patients' conduct. One of the main trends in gout eulogies was to contrast the luxuriously living sick with the healthy, poor and hardworking people who lived in the countryside in eternal penury. Rural folk, who satisfied their thirst with water, withstood famine and dressed in modest clothes, were hardly ever troubled by gout. The compilation of texts entitled *Dissertationes de laudibus et effectibus podagrae* (1715, pp. 14–15) listed renowned kings (King Asa who had arthritis; Agesilaus, the lame king of Sparta; Ptolemaeus), emperors (Galba, Severus, the Byzantine emperor Nicephorus) and popes (Honorius IV, Aeneas Sylvius or Pius II) as famous gout patients. The question of the social status of patients was raised in the same volume in a dialogue between a common man, Tityrus, and Jupiter. Tityrus, who represented the ordinary herdsman familiar from pastoral poetry, frequently was plagued by itch and fever but was never allowed to meet the goddess Podagra who dressed herself in jewels and golden necklaces, loved the court and kept her distance from ordinary and poor men (pp. 17–18).

That Gout had a special connection to highborn men made her noble, too. Ever since Lucian's mock-tragedies, Gout was deified in literature as a female goddess who commanded the world and especially rich men. For example, Georgius Bartholdus Pontanus (d. 1614) composed a dream vision of Gout's luxurious triumphal procession, *Triumphus Podagrae* (1605). In the poem the poet was taken to the valley of Tempe, where the queen Gout was parading among silver tables, golden utensils, jewels, heaps of delicacies brought from all over the world and gifts offered by other gods. The procession in her honour, probably parodying classical triumphs and royal entrées or imitating Apuleius' famous procession of Isis, included personified vices (Gula, Ebrietas), pleasures (Ludus, Risus), patients with distorted limbs, the playing of a lyre with trembling fingers and resemblance to the Horatian Chimera figure, a rich pharmacy, and servants such as Ischia, Arthritis, Chiragra, Mentagra, Nephritis and other diseases. The queen of the world was herself completely covered with gold and jewels and praised with a long hymn of adoration, sung by satyrs and bacchants, extolling her power as a moderator and teacher of good habits (1619, pp. 224–7).[17]

The Gout goddess's divine ancestry became a commonplace in a number of Neo-Latin texts on gout. It was brought out, for example, by Johannes Carnarius in his university speech *De podagrae laudibus oratio* (in Dornau 1619, 2: 219–24). Following the structure of Erasmus's *Moria* and the recognisable pattern of serious encomia, which began with the person's honourable origin, Carnarius dealt with the goddess's birth, family relationships and upbringing. Gout was born of Bacchus and Venus, the god and goddess whose gifts were dear to all Gout's patients (pp. 220–1). The anonymous *Podagraegraphia*, recounting the same origin, also noted certain family resemblances: from her father, Gout had inherited trembling hands and an insecure gait; from her mother, a predilection for wealthy men (pp. 224–5 [234–5]). In Carnarius's words, the baby Gout was nursed by Methe and Acratia, two nymphs and maids of Silenus and Venus; her servants included – with significant epithets – fat Polyphagia, sleepy Philypnia with thick eye lids, limping Misoponia, and Philedonia, bedecked with garlands and surrounded by floral perfumes (p. 221). In *Podagraegraphia* the same serving maids were mentioned, with elaborate epithets: Methe was from *Trunckenhausen*, Acratia from *unmessingen*, Polyphagia's cheeks were as thick as a flautist's and her belly protruded like the bellies of Hungarian cows (p. 226 [236]). The full adoring company in both Carnarius's speech and in *Podagraegraphia* included the chorus of Epicureans, maenads, satyrs and families called Weinheld or Sweinhard. In the same way, Erasmus's Moria was accompanied by a retinue of immoral abstractions, including selfishness, absentmindedness, laziness, hangover and various carnal pleasures.

The tale of Gout's family and entourage was usually followed by a description of her vast empire, which encompassed every place in the world, especially the palaces of rich men and the luxurious dining halls of pontifical courts, priests and abbots. Therefore, Balde called Gout the disease of kings and the King of diseases (1661, question 1). Carnarius objected to those who refused to count her among the goddesses on the grounds that no shrine or temple had ever been dedicated to her as had been to Febris, for instance. Just as Erasmus's Moria had emphasised her omnipotence, in Carnarius's view the whole world was Gout's sanctuary and she was celebrated everywhere (p. 222). *Podagraegraphia* claimed that Gout avoided infertile Lapland, the arid Arabian region, desert islands, caves and wild forests, since she needed fertile soil in which to flourish (p. 225 [235]). Thus, her hometown was in Nyssa, from where her father Bacchus came and the place of origin of many luxurious items, delicate fruits, precious jewels, spices and perfumes. The author stressed that Gout abhorred all forms of poverty, poor cottages, ordinary domestic animals like sheep with two teeth, the stench arising from swine's dunghills and simple tools designed for manual work. Instead, she preferred urban delicacies, glorious buildings and artfully decorated items like swords that were not meant for practical work (p. 226 [236]). She detested quotidian, around-the-clock work and stress, calling them her greatest enemies.

Podagraegraphia grew into a long attack against all forms of luxury, comparing luxurious living to swine and providing long lists of roasted dishes, meats, fishes and different wines that the rich man desired and that surpassed the delicacies offered to the gods themselves. The rich man's exclusive taste continuously demanded new culinary experiences, which the patient himself excogitated while lying down and counting flies. His friends were at pains to send new ingredients to him from abroad, and his wife struggled in the kitchen preparing new dishes, meanwhile suffering from insomnia caused by his constant demands for novelty (p. 239). The contrast between hardworking but poor people and those who earned great amounts of money simply by sitting or lying on their couches was elaborated upon in great detail. The caricature of the poor but healthy peasant depicted him as eating merely to survive, exercising his body through hard work, dressing in rags and stuffing his shoes with hay to keep his toes warm (p. 249).

Often retold was the fable of the travels of the spider and gout, which also introduced gout as the malady of the rich. Pantaleon Candidus (1540–1608), an Austrian theologian, poet and historiographer, who wrote Aesopian tales in verse, dedicated one poem to these two figures (1619, p. 229). Arachne the spider once lived with a rich man and filled every corner of his house with her webs. At the same time, Gout had taken up lodging in a poor man's cottage, but soon she realised that she did not feel welcome in his modest life, watching him eat black bread and sleep on a hard bed. When the spider's webs were repeatedly destroyed by the serving maids with their brooms, the two travellers decided to exchange lodgings, which made them both happy: Gout was entertained by the rich man's soft pillows and delicacies, whereas the spider had no trouble living peacefully in the poor man's hut.[18]

A similar anecdote entitled *Podagrae hospitium* by Jacobus Pontanus described how Gout once travelled in a woman's guise in the countryside (1619a, p. 224, quoting Jovianus Pontanus's *Bellaria Attica*). The dirty and flimsy shacks and small habitations, covered with spiders' webs, surrounded by simple farmer's tools and the reeking dunghills of cattle, did not please her. Therefore, she changed course for town, seeking leisure; there she found a pleasant house, which belonged to Otium and where people were dancing and a banquet was being celebrated. The inhabitants appealed to her, devoted as they were to drinking; they appeared somnolent and had no obligations to work. Worries, work, sobriety and abstinence were all barred from the house, into which Gout then settled down with deep pleasure, and said, "This is my home, this is my country" (*Haec domus, haec patria*).

These stories were overtly morally critical in constantly stressing that Gout was absent from poor homes. This was confirmed by the prescriptions given for a cure. Balde relied in his satirical prescriptions on expert healers' advice, according to which the most efficient remedies for gout were the three Graces – Inedia, Inedia and Inedia. However, Balde also noted that not all Hippocratic doctors believed in fasting or in complete abstinence from food; rather the Pythagoreans suggested the following honest diet: "As the first course, serve peas and vegetables; second, vegetables and peas; third, vegetables with peas; and fourth, peas with vegetables" (1661, question 24). Balde also elaborated on the Roman satirists' reminders that the disease should be treated at the first sign, in the very cradle, before the calf has grown to an adult bull (1661, poem 82).

Disease eulogies aspired to change the balance between the noble and the poor and thereby to remind one that true virtue did not depend on wealth or distinguished ancestry. The balancing act was realised not only in the fact that gout attacked rich men who became poor through illness, but also in the way gout patients – now understood as poor and pitiable because of their illness – were honoured and esteemed even over noblemen. Several gout eulogies (Pirckheimer 2002, §45–6; *Podagraegraphia*, p. 256) noted how the crowd made way for the patient in the streets; he was allowed to sit in the presence of kings, his wishes were always granted, he was served special delicacies and whatever else he wished to eat. Friends and servants were always around, and the sense of awe was discerned in the splendour of the palaces gout usually inhabited. In his *Podagrae encomium*, Cardano observed that the gout patient rode while others walked, so that Maximianus Stampa was riding a mule while Prince Alphonsus was on foot (1619, p. 218). The patient was carried in a gout chair like the noble Romans, or as Balde noted, like idols and images of gods that black African priests carried while singing (1661, poem 16). Owing to their disease, Brazilian tyrants and other barbaric rulers hardly ever walked on their own feet, but were carried on the shoulders of their slaves while happily chewing on sweet herbs. Thus, it was nearly divine just to sit, to be adored like a god and not to howl in pain, since gods do not complain. Gout and her patients were thus full of majesty (*Dissertationes de laudibus et effectibus podagrae*, p. 111).

Changes discerned in the social hierarchy caused by gout served satirical criticism, which questioned the true nobility of the rich and reminded them that the poor and humble could exceed them in many ways. *Podagraegraphia* (p. 230) noted that poverty, when appearing with a just mind, was not the worst of evils, since true evil was always something dishonourable (a claim frequently repeated in paradoxical eulogies). Disease images were thus bound up with those socio-economic biases that were so dear to satirical moralists. The gulf between the rich and the poor was maintained and the distance between different classes was drawn in the area of disease as well. Even though the lower classes often fell victims to epidemics and malnutrition, in satires the rich man was usually the more seriously ill and did not enjoy a higher life expectancy. Diseases like gout were used to describe his alleged immorality in particular, and hence, disease eulogies acquired satirically critical tones.

Enduring pain like a Stoic

Gout was praised, because in her divine and unquestionable power she could affect the power of the rich and punish them for their moral transgressions. Punitive satires gave detailed accounts of violent changes discerned in the patient's distorted body, which also functioned as satirical warnings and threats. The satirists revelled at his desperation and useless prayers for mercy. The Chorus in Lucian's *Tragodopodagra* sang of the excruciating pains that afflicted virtually every limb as if by sharp weapons and boasted of how the luckless men lay shrieking as attacks tortured them (119–24).

These passages inspired many imitators in the early modern age. In one ode, Jesuit poet Lieven De Meyere (1655–1730), for instance, deplored the creeping pains burning in his innermost being, which neither his heroic protests, his visiting friends nor the soothing ointments of the mythical surgeon Machaon could ease. Sisyphus and Tantalus were considered mere poets' dreams when compared with so grave a torment as gout, called here the one sole punishment for all.[19] De Meyere's poem was elegiac in tone, but a satirical Neo-Latin example describing a similar painful condition was the dialogue *Morbidi duo* between a gout patient and a gall stone or kidney stone patient composed by Jacobus Pontanus (1542–1626), a Jesuit and professor of rhetoric, grammar and poetry at Augsburg and Dillingen.[20] The short dialogue opened with loud lamentations from the two sufferers, each complaining about his fate and assessing it as worse than the condition caused by any other disease (1619b, pp. 214–15). As in Lucian's dialogue, the gout patient compared himself with the famous convicts of ancient mythology, Tantalus and Sisyphus, and their agonies. Whereas epileptic, paralysed and lethargic patients had hopes of regaining their health, gout offered no such prospects. Neither were the pains alleviated by medication; all remedies turned out to be useless. The kidney stone patient wailed even more desperately, regretting that he had failed to abstain from cheese, milk, turnips, and fatty and salted meat. His complaint continued with a long list of prohibited foods and drinks and detailed descriptions of how pastries and other delicacies filled the body parts with crude fluids and aggravated the internal organs. The descriptions benefited from contemporary medical ideas about causes of the disease, that is, overeating, but in the name of satirical punishment, the symptoms' distress was emphasised as was the self-acquired unhealthy condition.

The gout patient deplored the fact that he resembled a living corpse rather than a human being, whereas the kidney stone patient said he felt like small knives were cutting his flesh as the stones travelled through the veins. The gout patient reminded him that larger kidney stones could be surgically operated on, whereas his own disease could not be relieved by any such measures unless both legs were amputated. This gave the kidney stone patient reason to recall the screams of horror from two surgical patients, one of them having died simply from pain. But the kidney stone patient thought that many healthy but poor men would gladly change places with the gouty man in order to have the advantages of his life, including friends, well-prepared food, soft pillows, leisure time and freedom from all duties and cares. Further advantages of gout were that when the body was weak, the mind became stronger; the excess fluids that otherwise conglomerate and are deposited in the internal organs were now directed to the extreme body parts, which increased overall health. Furthermore, gout taught many virtues: the patient hardly ever suffered from ambition, arrogance or envy. When the gout patient grumbled that other diseases had similar favourable effects as well, the kidney stone patient once again contradicted him, saying that other diseases were usually either lethal or had no let-up in the torments and thus hardly offered time for learned leisure, as did gout. At the end of the dialogue the discussants moved onto a meta-literary plane, mentioning earlier praises and Lucian's disease eulogies. The only remedy against these diseases was a moderate mind. The text closed with reference to Seneca, saying that even in distress, the moderate mind gave men consolation.

The dialogue reflected the satirical pleasure taken in the punishment of the victims and ridiculed their complaints. The Lucianic spirit of mocking serious suffering was clearly involved. But gout was also appropriate for playful ethical discussions, the reason being that, as an extremely troublesome and painful disease, it offered the Stoic-minded moralists a perfect case whereby to test one's ability to endure pain courageously. When recording voices of pain in his *Solatium podagricorum*, Balde asserted that complete silence was not required, but mindless yelling reminiscent of madly howling wild boars or bellowing bulls did not suit a wise man, for whom suitable voices of suffering were muffled sighs, murmurs and whispers (1661, poems 39–41). These bespoke his self-restraint and dignity and separated him from brute beasts. The mourner's noisy over-reaction to a small loss of money was also ridiculed in Juvenal's satire 13, which is an ironic consolation (Braund 1997, p. 74; Morford 1973). Petrarch also stressed that the wise man should remain tranquil in the face of suffering and never to complain (McClure 1990, p. 41).

The screams of pain were a concrete reminder of the Stoic discussions about how men should respond to suffering. In his ironic consolatory epistle, Seneca had advised that there is a certain propriety and moderation to be observed even in the act of grieving (99.21; Wilson 1997, p. 58). People may generally assume that a crippling and painful condition was exclusively an evil that impeded happiness and the best possible life. In his *Epistulae* (78.6) Seneca mentioned three elements – fear of death, physical pain and interruption of pleasure – that were thought to accompany every disease and were considered reasons for great suffering in sick people's lives. However, Seneca also maintained that blindness, crippling or other physical afflictions did not alone render a man unhappy (92.22). In his epistle dealing with the healing power of the mind over physical pain, Seneca questioned the negative impact of disease on human life, arguing, for example, that seemingly unfavourable diseases can teach men to perceive the true value of things (78.7–9). He denied the negativity of suffering on the grounds that it was often made endurable when attacks of pain were interrupted and had intervals of rest. Significantly, gout was used here as an example of such a disease. Likewise, Epicurus, who endured a diseased bladder and an ulcerated stomach, had claimed that physical pain was not a source of unhappiness, since an intense pain was usually brief and chronic pain could be made endurable (66.47). Although disease checked the body's pleasures, in Seneca's words it did not do away with them but excited them and made them more rewarding. Moreover, to do without pleasure was in fact something the good man should aspire to, and the most important pleasures, which were those of the mind, no disease (or doctor) could abolish (78.22).[21]

Pain and disease were not real evils, since evil was measured in moral terms. In *De oratore* (2.342, 346), Cicero claimed that good looks and physical strength were external gifts that did not in themselves contain any real grounds for praise. Virtues were revealed in the correct use of their benefits, since it was in the realm of action and making choices that virtues were manifested.[22] In these discussions physical strength or health was considered a quality that the person himself could not affect, and therefore, strength was not related to personal virtue. Likewise in the Stoic view, neither poverty nor illness could affect a man who possessed virtue and who was able to transcend the body's trivial demands. Diseases were regarded as external or indifferent things that could not harm the balanced inner self of the wise man who was indifferent to fortune and transcended both pleasure and pain. His attitude secured his freedom, since he was no longer enslaved by their tyranny, but mastered them and himself (Seneca, *De vita beata* 4.4–5; *De consolatione ad Marciam* 10.1). Moreover, since virtue was made manifest in its dealings with things like sickness, pain or poverty, diseases were useful in presenting courage, heroic endurance of pain and self-control in difficult situations. As Seneca noted, there was room for virtue even on the sick bed (*Epistulae* 78.20–1; 67.4). Enduring suffering and conquering pain were also traditional heroic goals in literary genres such as the epic and in poetry that either lamented the pains caused by disease[23] or extolled them as a sweet and pleasurable experience.[24]

Paradoxical encomia were stimulated by these philosophical commonplaces and thoughts of pain, suffering and disease and were sometimes playful restatements of the themes of Stoic paradoxes in general, which emphasised the freedom of the human spirit from the environment and worldly bonds.[25] Latin philosophical works, especially the second Book of Cicero's *Tusculanae disputationes* and Seneca's moral epistles to Lucilius, were frequently quoted in early modern disease eulogies that reflected the Stoic value system. In his praise of gout, Carnarius recalled how the Stoics, Epicureans and other ancient philosophers like Socrates had despised even severe pain as insignificant. Carnarius recalled an anecdote about the Stoic Posidonius, who had courageously endured paroxysms of gout in the joints and argued from his sickbed that the pain tortured him in vain, since he would never acknowledge it as an evil (p. 223; Cicero, *Tusc.* 2.25.61). With its reference to Cicero and ancient philosophy in general, *Podagraegraphia* noted that death and disease were neither intolerable nor the worst evils, just as old age did not necessarily make life troublesome nor was an innocent exile infamous (pp. 230, 245). An evil was by definition something dishonourable, whereas diseases were merely indifferent. Thus, physical pain was distinguished from suffering; even a courageous man sensed pain, but he refused to suffer from it.

Balde, for his part, wrote his *Solatium podagricorum* entirely in Stoic terms, playfully mixing Stoic consolation with his writing. In his words, he had adopted the Stoic standpoint for the simple reason that the Peripatetic perambulation in the Academia did not suit men with ailing feet. He called his learned and dignified addressees "Archpodagric heroes," to whom he offered the Archstoics' solid food, not the honey-coated sweets that boys loved (1661, question 42). Balde advised patients to despise and laugh at pain and rejoice in the severe condition of man (poem 37). The inflexibility and defiance characteristic of the Stoics was also evident in his words urging the disease to burn, slash and excruciate the body, meanwhile assuring that the mind would remain unmoved and invincible (poem 86): "A blind fire rages like a tempest inside, but I will not complain. It tears me, but I will not complain. It carves me, but the pain will never force a sigh to burst from my lips." A Stoic (and an Epicurean) commonplace was also reflected in his words that denied the pain as real or an evil; it was rather merely the image of pain and an opinion originating in the minds of ignorant men.

In consolatory literature, philosophy was usually recommended as an aid to coping with pain (Braund 1997, p. 75; Erskine 1997, p. 38). Thus, in Balde's view, the best therapy against gout was Stoic philosophy, and the body should be literally soothed with the wise man's words (1661, poem 43):

> When the furious ardour penetrates the body, put Cleanthes under your neck, cover your breast with Zeno and big Cebes, hide Seneca and Thrasea under your pillow, let your feet rest on Epictetus and let your body be doctored by the Phrygian. If the pain forces you to utter a cry that is not worthy of tranquil ears and if your tongue foams with shameful saliva, cover your face with Speusippus and invest the mouth with hard bits and a Pythagorean bolt, so that an unworthy voice shall not pass from your lips and spoil your immaculate reputation.

The books of learned men were remedies that helped the patient to overcome his grief, but Balde's concrete way of using philosophy as therapy is deeply ironic; he seemed to have a whole Stoic library in his use. Later Balde advised the patient to drain Cleanthes' effervescent cup, which contained tonic with a strong taste of sulphur, salt and old metal (poem 85). Balde thus advocated a slightly different therapy than Persius (5.63–4), who had suggested the seed of Cleanthes be sown in the patient's scrubbed ears. Balde represented Christian Neo-Stoicism, which had become a prominent mode of thinking in the Baroque period (Schäfer 1976, pp. 215–18), but always preserved his characteristic irony and parody in his discussions of the good life.

In disease eulogies the wise man was advised to rise above the pain so that it would not severely affect his life. He could thereby prove that he was not bound to his body. Diseases were regarded as having positive, active effects on man's life, teaching him good values and eventually strengthening his intellectual, spiritual and moral capacities. In the same way Erasmus's Moria had argued that she made all men happy and rendered their pleasures more rewarding. Instead of seeing bodily vexations as harmful, punishing or at best bearable, early modern authors also praised them as preferable to many other kinds of suffering or even to good health, which was widely seen as a requisite for the good life. Balde began his consolation by saying that even doctors regarded gout as a hateful, horrible, wretched and incurable disease, a definition which he then challenged (1661, p. 1). Changing names and attributes commonly given to diseases was one strategy for re-evaluating the harm they caused. Balde's list of gout's attributes reflected conceptions that he regarded as false:

> Common folk call gout a patrician malady; patricians call it thirsty and delicate; Peripatetic philosophers call it Stoic; Stoics call it sedentary;

> all medical doctors call it hateful; some, stubborn and intractable; the Galenics, difficult; the Empirics, knotty; the Chymics, tartaric; some patients, infernal (*Tartareus*); the poets, human, ingenious and insolent; orators, consular and worthy of curulian chairs. (question 1)

Later in his consolation Balde characterised gout as a knotty teacher (poem 26), an inner advisor and a domestic Chiron (poem 31).

Thus, owing to its morally and intellectually elevating effects, gout was paradoxically a salutary disease (*morbus salutaris*) or, when encouraging Christian virtues or considered an affliction sent by God, a blessed malady (Carnarius, p. 223; *Podagraegraphia*, p. 245). Some texts, like the second part of the *Podagraegraphia*, turned into downright moralising and, by quoting Christian sentences, reminded its readers that the constant vexations and trials were chosen and sent by God who thereby prepared men to ascend to his kingdom. The texts attacked leisure as the source of sins, physical illness and loss of honour.[26]

That diseases were no less useful than philosophy in assisting in the process of developing virtue was also noted in Erasmus's letter to Willibald Pirckheimer and published as a preface to Erasmus's edition of St John Chrysostom's *De sacerdotio* in 1525 (Tomarken 1990, pp. 47–8). In Erasmus's words (1619, p. 202), if philosophy meant preparation for and the practice of death, as it was with Socrates in *Phaedo* (81a), then kidney stones, as a meditation on death, were the highest philosophy. Ironically, kidney stones were celebrated, since they trained men to endure pain and taught them how to accept death so that they learned not to be afraid of it and even more, came to long for it in order to be released from the annoying disease called *ipsa mors*, death itself. In his epistle (54), Seneca had praised asthma by using similar arguments: he was no longer afraid of death, because for so long he had been prepared down to the last breath. He compared lack of breath to a continued last gasp; physicians had called it "practicing how to die". Similarly, an early sixteenth-century Italian poet Matteo Francesi praised the cough, saying that by keeping him awake at night it gave him time to meditate and create poems (Tomarken 1990, p. 94).

The blessings of gout

The philosophical and rhetorical traditions met in early modern paradoxical eulogies. The rhetorical background was reflected in their legal imagery, in several gout eulogies which were situated in court before an opposing party and the judge – a similar trial scene was found in

Erasmus's *Moria*. Personified Gout acted as an advocate to defend herself against common opinion, rumours, impugnment of her reputation and false accusations presented against her by the crowd. One should remember that false beliefs are also the main target of philosophy. Helius Eobanus Hessus (1488–1540), a famous poet and professor at Erfurt and Nuremberg, translated a German poem into Latin as *Podagrae ludus* (1537), and this poem, together with Pirckheimer's *Apologia seu Podagrae laus* and the second part of *Podagraegraphia,* were good examples of the characteristic courtroom defence.

In court Pirckheimer's Gout argued that people tended to regard her as a source of many pains and evils, although it was the patients' own immoral behaviours that had caused the disease. Equally misplaced, in Gout's opinion, would be charges made by those who deliberately committed suicide by fire and afterwards blaming the fire, or those who drowned themselves and then blamed the water for their death. Using a typical courtroom device, Gout shifted the blame to the opposing party, the patients, claiming that their own culpable acts and morally depraved, leisurely lifestyles had actually caused her deeds (2002, §25–8). Pirckheimer's Gout performed her job reluctantly, but even though the extravagant luxury annoyed her, she was forced to act upon the patients against her will. Defences required proofs, and the visible signs of the patients' own culpability included drunkenness, hangovers and constant drinking. The pale faces, green skin colour, twisted gait and overall unhealthy appearance also were clear signs of inveterate bad living and guilt (§29; *Podagraegraphia*, p. 254).

Pirckheimer's Gout also gave a list of the physical signs that she caused and that were used as arguments against her: she metamorphosed the patient by diluting his blood, changing the skin colour, weakening the life force, causing insomnia, clouding the eyes, slowing down the movements and turning the whole body round-shouldered and weak (§64). However, Gout protested against these accusations by re-interpreting the signs and arguing that the inflicted body could be read in her defence, since clearly she focused on the physical and hence, inferior, animal side. Gout triumphed over her prosecutors by asserting that while attacking the vile flesh and mortal body, she ultimately cured the soul and strengthened the spirit. Thus, she served human development no less if she were practicing philosophy, theology and legislation. This argument was followed by a list of the inconveniences caused by the body, including unhealthy appetites, passions and other diseases of the mind (*animi egritudines*), which ensued from insatiable physical desires and prevented men from resting or from concentrating on the contemplative life (§65). These ill effects were not only harmful to individual morality, but also affected entire societies, when personal desires led to larger quarrels, wars, crimes, murders, revolutions, thefts and fires (cf. *Podagraegraphia*, p. 260).

One of the major argumentative strategies in these eulogies was thus to confirm the philosophical (or Platonic) opposition between body and mind. In this antagonism, the body was an enemy on the way to moral and intellectual perfection. Likewise, in Petrarch's *De remediis utriusque fortunae* (II.84, *De podagra*), Reason confronted foot with heart and head and considered aching feet a minor problem. Cicero also noted in his *Tusculans* (2.19.44) that Philoctetes' pain was not severe, since it was only in the foot. In his *Solatium podagricorum* Balde seemed to elaborate on these ideas. Balde reminded the patient who moaned about his aching foot that his mind was still free to reach the heavens and advised him to disdain the extreme body part. In Balde's words, it was mindless to long to run when the patient was not a tightrope walker, athlete or horse; serving boys were in the household for that function (1661, poem 11). The brain and virtuous speech were the best things a man could have. Homer, who was blind and crippled, did not, in Balde's view, travel across countries, and yet he became so famous worldwide that seven towns competed for the honour of being identified as his place of birth (poem 65). Balde advised the patient to dismiss foolish ideas about running around the stadium; it was better to rely on virtue than on the feet; moreover, only fools despised quietude or prayed for something useless or shameful. The desire to be able to run was considered as absurd as wanting a horse's tail, a harpy's nails or a bear's frantic jaws (poems 16–20). By describing the patient's groundless complaint of not being able to walk along muddy streets, the poems demanded recognition of the true value of things. Balde also reminded the Christian of his mortality, the vanity of all earthly things and of earthly tribulations of every kind, which could not be controlled by humans. But Balde's way of underlining the human condition and the utmost vanity of the mundane world was always humorous and satirical, as is seen here: humanity epitomised in the painful gouty foot that, however, helped men to attain true virtue, since it kept them from touching the vile earth.

Sometimes gout benefited the body, such as when it caused loss of weight during a long illness or purified the body of excess fluids (Pirckheimer 2002, §68). Balde cleverly compared thick bodily humours with clear poetic fountains, saying that such stagnated fluids offered no inspiration to poets (1661, poem 81). Paradoxical eulogies did not argue for the simple inferiority or uselessness of the body, since the body could, by taking the form of headaches, drunkenness, sleepiness or disease, affect the mind in a positive way. But the final conclusion was not against the conventional view that the mind commanded the body, since the afflicted body was always inferior to the mind, even though body could help mind to achieve perfection. As the author of *Podagraegraphia* put it, the mind was to the body what a mechanism is to a clock, a rider to a horse, a smith to a hammer, or a fire to an oven – it used the body's limbs as its instruments (p. 232).

Another conventional rhetorical strategy by which Gout defended her case was to argue that the disadvantages she caused were far fewer than the benefits she afforded human life. Most of the benefits were generated by the patient's perpetual immobility and enforced leisure. In Balde's words, gout patients were immobile like the gods and affixed to their beds like polyps to stones or mushrooms to rocks (1661, poem 19). The conventional assumption about the sick man's isolation and loneliness was refuted, when Pirckheimer's Gout included among the benefits a comfortable couch on which to rest, frequent visits by well-wishing friends, gifts received, jokes told at the sickbed and the laughter often heard from patients' homes (§43). Laughter was known to have a healing effect on men as did poetry. Balde related that musician and poet Richard Mamphulus ordered Ovid's fables to be read aloud to him when seized by a paroxysm of gout (1661, poem 58). Another patient, Leonard Crinallus Veldkirchensis, used Lucan's *Pharsalia* for consolation, since the war scenes reminded him that his condition was not unbearable (poem 60). Erasmus also noted that gout's misery was alleviated by fables told by friends (1619, p. 202); earlier, Seneca had claimed that the cheering words of his friends and their conversation at the bedside greatly improved his health (*Epistulae* 78.4). When Roman verse satire employed the common sickbed scene, the visitors were motivated by hopes of inheritance, but here disease allowed the patient to be accompanied by a selected band of like-minded men, as if in a philosophical school, which supplied a private, social setting for practising the philosophical life. The social calls were occasions for discussion, amusement and showing friendship.[27]

The philosophical opposition between the contemplative life and the active life was maintained in many disease eulogies. That the patient was not able to move was a perfect excuse for not taking any political action or participating in public decision-making. Thus, gout made the patient's life easier and liberated him from all strenuous duties. The excuse was already noted in Martial's epigram (7.39), with reference to a man called Caelius who, tired of early morning calls and saluting wealthy patrons, pretended to have gout. Balde mentioned *pseudopodagrici* who simulated gout paroxysms in order to enjoy rest and soft pillows; they had an avid desire merely to sit peacefully (1661, poem 27). Disease eulogies thus interpreted the condition of being left alone positively, in contrast to the conventional view of solitude as some of the greatest miseries of sickness. Gout eulogies repeatedly stressed that, when forced to stay at home and live a solitary life, the patient avoided not only obligations but also many other social inconveniences and quarrels. Pirckheimer's Gout saw that she protected people from dangers and accidents when they were unable to sail, hunt or make war (§52). They escaped shipwrecks, accidental shooting, wild beasts, fist-fights, false ambitions, arrogance and especially the three chief vices – anger, drunkenness and shameful desire.

Of the ancient Stoics, Seneca had placed the heaviest emphasis on the contemplative life. If there were three kinds of life, as he argued in *De otio* (7.1), each devoted either to pleasure, contemplation or action, then diseases were useful in the life that focused on contemplation.[28] Absolute solitude was difficult to achieve in normal life, but diseases guaranteed a human being isolated circumstances and the pleasures of retirement that were beneficial to moral and intellectual improvement. In his epistles Seneca had advised Lucilius to withdraw from the daily life of men and affairs and argued that even though the body was hampered by ill health, the soul was still able to work (7; 78.20).

Likewise, the paradoxical authors argued that the patient suffering from gout was forced to mend his lifestyle.[29] Hence, he had a lot of time and energy to devote to self-scrutiny and learning, especially about such crucial issues as health and suffering, all without any interference from the outside. Diseased leisure did not mean sloth or idleness, although no public service or participation in social affairs was involved, but a *vita contemplativa* that celebrated isolation from the secular world. Prison was paradoxically praised in the same sense and used as a setting by Boethius in his *De consolatione philosophiae*, where the prisoner, on the point of death, was forced to wrestle with eternal questions.[30] Illness in its isolation formed a desirable and liberating asylum for the patient, since it separated him from the mad world. This view – that man was closer to reality when he was withdrawn from the physical world – was a commonplace in Stoic contemplative literature (Relihan 2007, p. 38).

Pirckheimer's Gout thus insisted that the enforced sedentary lifestyle was the cause of many good things in a man's life, since patients learned more while sitting than in running or dancing (§54–62). Patients had time to learn languages and study the liberal arts. They even acquired special skills, such as weather observation: their weather forecasts were exceptionally reliable, for their joints were sensitive to its variations. Their expertise also included medicine, since during the long treatment the patients became familiar with numerous medical drugs and herbs (cf. Cardano 1619, p. 218; *Podagraegraphia*, pp. 258–9). In her own words, Gout caused the suffering patient to realise the folly of leading a luxurious life, which was the primary cause of the illness, and thus she made him change his lifestyle. Although the body and the flesh suffered in the gout attack, the mind became free and healthy (Cardano 1619, p. 217, *in morbo sanior quam bona valetudine*). Balde also recalled Aristotle's saying, "by sitting men become wise" (1661, poem 66), as well as the words of a famous gout patient, Enea Silvio Piccolomini – "I have astrological feet and hands" (poem 54). Sick leave had produced many learned texts in history: Cardano noted that we owe many interesting books to gout (1619, pp. 217–18). It was well known that Ennius claimed in one of his satirical fragments that he wrote only when attacked by gout, and Balde also mentioned other authors and encyclopaedic writers who owed their inspiration to gout (1661, poems 61–2). Thus, Pirckheimer's personified Gout claimed that she was not to be blamed, despite what most people seemed to think.

Pirckheimer's Gout also claimed to improve the patient's character by curing serious vices, arrogance and ambition; the patient learned to be content with very little. Gout punished especially the three main vices that made a patient prone to this illness, namely, overeating, sexual excess and quick temper (§70–2). She also excused her at times rough treatment by comparing herself with medical doctors, who never hesitated to have recourse to the already familiar devices of fire and knife to improve their patients' condition – at least when all other healing efforts had failed (§80). As the virtues promoted by gout, Cardano listed chastity, piety, temperance, prudence, industriousness, moderation and constancy of mind (1619, p. 218). Gout also preserved men from vanity, useless thoughts, groundless fear and false hopes. It made pleasures stronger since they were rare – wine tasted better in the former patients' mouths. Gout not only inspired virtues but also religious faith by reminding human beings of their mortality and perishable conditions, accustomed them to frequent prayers and made them humble and devout. The vanity of human life was revealed to the patient when he discovered how transitory his physical strength was. The Christian perspective was also present in many disease eulogies; for example, Cardano claimed that no one was as thoughtful of the gods as a gout patient.

Gout thus resulted in many positive changes in character by binding the patient's feet and forcing him to be immobile. Carnarius (p. 222) and *Podagraegraphia* (p. 242) remarked that patients turned humble: when in his arrogance and prompted by his success in war Alexander the Great came to believe that he was the son of Jupiter, pain and battle wounds quickly proved him to be a son of Philip and softened his hard character. Likewise, an anonymous stubborn man, refusing to obey the precepts of philosophy and despising his friends' admonitions to be moderate, completely changed his life after a paroxysm of gout and soon excelled Diogenes in temperance, Socrates in wisdom and Xenocrates in chastity.

Disease also had amazing and crucial effects on intelligence: Hieron, the tyrant of Sicily, did not differ much from his idiot brother before his disease, but afterwards he became the closest friend and patron of the famous poets Simonides, Pindar and Bacchylides. Carnarius remarked (p. 222) that a similar development was noted in Ptolemaeus II and in Theagenes, the Athenian senator. Likewise, Straton the athlete once lived luxuriously, but after his disease he won the first prize in four major Greek sports competitions. And Balde, when responding to why gout patients were more intelligent than others, said (1661, question 37): "Their head is more serene. The thick vapours that usually obscured the brain were now directed downwards to the supporting pillars of the human body. The same effect can be discerned when the east wind blows and clears the mountains, suppressing the mists and rainy clouds down to the valley." By helping the mind to achieve the ideal state of serenity, gout thus improved and transformed the character no less than philosophy or perhaps even the Christian faith.

Gout was also defended by comparing its effects with those of other diseases, a topos in gout eulogies (Carnarius, p. 223; *Podagraegraphia*, pp. 243, 245, 255). Gout differed from other diseases in that it did not afflict such vital organs as the brain, heart or liver, but was satisfied with attacking an external and most insignificant part of the human body, the foot. It did not harm people's rational faculty or memory as did other diseases; neither did it cause insanity or desperation. In *Dissertationes de laudibus et effectibus podagrae* (pp. 37, 72, 78), Gout's modesty was also explained by the fact that it attacked the humblest part of the human body. There was also embedded a wordplay on the humble character (*humilis*) and the humours which filled the feet with gout. In fact, gout improved health by directing the excess fluids into the extreme body parts and thereby preserved the patient from serious ill-effects of over-nutrition. In the same vein Plutarch had recorded it as an encouraging symptom if the disease turned to the less vital parts of the body; significantly, this medical comparison was used in his discussion of the progress in virtue ("How a man may become aware of his progress in virtue", *Moralia* 84A). Authors like Cardano stressed that, compared with other diseases, gout was well behaved. Whereas other diseases were often chronic and cruel to the patient, subjecting them to continuous, excruciating pain, causing desperation and leaving people without hope of recovery, Gout, by contrast, always permitted relief during intervals when she produced no symptoms. Pirckheimer's Gout also justified her morally responsible conduct by emphasising that unlike other diseases, she treated people equally, be they kings, priests or princes, noble or ignoble (§40). On the other hand, she was called peace loving, since she attacked only men in their full vigour while sparing women, eunuchs, children, old people and others who were weak (*Podagraegraphia*, p. 240; Cardano 1619, p. 217). This revealed Gout's generous character and showed that she had a firm sense of justice.

The list of gout's virtues was supplemented by comparing her with other specific diseases: she was not shameful or repulsive, as were leprosy, the itch or venereal diseases, nor was she contagious as were phthisis, the plague or opthalmia (Cardano 1619, pp. 218–19). Neither did she cause annoying symptoms such as wounds, coughs, vomiting or diarrhoea, but behaved decently and had a pure character. Medical literature knew the concept of benevolent disease (*morbus benignus*), which did not cause any other serious symptoms except for those that were its own (Sennert 1628, p. 194); gout clearly belonged to this category. Likewise, Balde reminded of the gentleness of gout compared with furious diseases of the brain or kidney stones that recalled Sisyphus' suffering or the erotic horrors of venereal pus (1661, poem 52). It was also good to remember the passions of Christ or the tortures of the Underworld and not exaggerate one's own ailments (poem 84).

The virtues Cardano attributed to gout were identical with those enumerated in serious praises of kings and rulers (1619, pp. 216–19). These included modesty, since gout took its name from the humble but by no means dirty member, the human foot; honesty and uprightness, since she made open attacks without using tricks or deceiving the patient; the sense of justice and temperance, since she afflicted all men, kings, emperors and priests alike, but only as long as the man could stand her attacks, these being followed by a short pause to alleviate the patient's suffering; gentleness, since she did not harm people who were already poor; courage, since she fought doctors and medicine fearlessly; and military power, since she occupied and took full command of the whole body and expelled other diseases.[31]

Dissertationes de laudibus et effectibus podagrae also argued that gout was not extravagant and did not run around like an Olympic runner but stayed firmly in one place, usually at home (pp. 43, 61). The author compared gout with a beautiful rose: she made the feet reddish – the blush was also a sign of bashfulness – and the pains she caused were likened to thorns (p. 84). Gout was moderate; at a banquet she was satisfied with mere spiritual nourishment (with a pun on "spirits") (p. 98). She was decent and possessed chastity, this being proved by the fact that she never allowed anyone to touch even the feet (p. 143). Gout was innocent too, considering that the patient was lying on his bed like an infant in a cradle (p. 151).

In early modern moral discourse, diseases were thus thought to have many advantages. First and foremost, they left the patient time for meditation because he was prevented from engaging in social activities and was thereby removed from the company of malicious men or the temptations of the outer world. Gout also enforced temperance and rendered the patient stronger than he was before the attack. And the pleasant remedies used against gout, including a moderate amount of sleep, some wine, music and wise companions, were not bad either (Tomarken 1990, p. 61). In his *Podagrae encomium*, Cardano thus even argued that his praise of gout did not fall into the category of paradoxical encomia, since gout was not evil but openly beneficial. His purpose was not to show his wit or eloquence in defending the indefensible or frivolous, but to point out in a serious manner the goodness of gout. Therefore Cardano's encomium has sometimes been taken as a serious treatise, but it belongs to satirical eulogies in the best tradition of the genre (Tomarken 1990, pp. 62–3).

Matthaeus Czanakius: in praise of the itch

In the sixteenth and seventeenth centuries, there were numerous speeches, essays and poems written to extol gout or blindness, but it was far more infrequent to praise scabies, the itch and scratching.[32] Visible signs of the itching – blisters, pustules and pimples – were hardly regarded as beautiful or worthy of aesthetic praise; they were associated with the ragged poor and rotten conditions and were often accompanied or caused by a host of biting lice, gnats and fleas. Yet it was the very association with such conditions that inspired paradoxical praises of the itch, since in satires the poor were usually virtuous and hard working. Thus, their diseases also had potentially positive moral significance. The poor were satisfied with little and their life was filled with constant vexation – epitomised by scratching – but for that very reason, scratching was virtuous. In the morality of satire, the road of vice was pleasant and easy but deceptive, whereas on the narrower and harder path of virtue pains, worries and diseases were encountered, yet this was the recommended route. Virtue was not achieved without toil and effort, and the itch became linked with these virtues. Here, the itch did not refer to people's diseased and immoral condition in general, as it did in the context of verse satire. For example, Casaubon (1780, p. 223) claimed that Juvenal's satires attacked people's scaly skin (*scabies scalpitur*), and Johann Lauremberg's (1590–1658) satirical verses endeavoured to scratch men's scabby hearts (*scabiosa corda*) with biting pepper and satirical salt (1684, p. 8). Rather it referred to a skin disease that caused ethically-elevating experiences. It was probably also associated with the irritation caused by venereal diseases, which were also known by the name scabies.[33]

Thus, Matthaeus M. Czanakius (Czanaki Máté, c. 1595–1630), a Hungarian doctor who had studied in Heidelberg and Bremen, wrote a noble praise of the itch in 1627, *Nobile scabiei encomium*. Like Pontanus's triumph of gout, Czanakius's paean was addressed to a large group of patients, to everyone suffering from itch in the noble republic of scabby people. Czanakius saw his work as continuing the tradition of Erasmus's *Moria*, and its purpose was to deal with the nature, origin and cure of the malady. The eulogy also had a link to certain philosophical discussions. In Plato's *Gorgias* (494), Callicles and Socrates playfully discussed whether pleasure acquired from any source whatsoever was good and valuable. Since an itching man's greatest desires were easily satisfied by scratching, Socrates ironically asked whether this satisfaction rendered his life happy. In *Philebus* (51c), the discussants mentioned the pleasure of scratching as a potential form of relief and pleasure that eased the pain caused by the itch. Itching also belonged to the impure and troublesome pleasures needing catharsis.[34] In his *De tranquillitate animi* (2.11–12), Seneca mentioned scabies when he dealt with the sick and restless mind: "Just as there are some sores which crave the hands that will hurt them and rejoice to be touched, and as a foul itch of the body delights in whatever scratches, exactly so, I would say, do these minds upon which, so to speak, desires have broken out like wicked sores find pleasure in toil and vexation" (trans. John W. Basore). Plutarch, for his part, compared a man who required stimulations of taste by odours to the itch, which required continual scratching ("Advice about keeping well", *Moralia* 126B). Right after this he argued that diseases did not take from us our enterprises or pastimes but our pleasures, and therefore infirmities allowed us to become philosophers.

Plato's anti-somatic words did not call for an acceptance of scratching as an ethical activity, but he used the itch as a parodically concrete example of a simple, pleasant activity. But in Czanakius's parodical treatment, the itch in fact did result in happiness, because by providing work against the temptations of idleness, it brought joy and encouraged many fundamental virtues. Praise of the itch thus contributed to that pervasive theme of disease eulogies, namely, the best possible life and ethical development was achieved through an illness.

Czanakius's preface and dedication to his essay included a typical satirical assessment, according to which the appearance of things was often deceptive and a glorious surface concealed serious vices. Czanakius claimed that people should not be judged by their clothing, since a dirty cloak could conceal wisdom, whereas thieves and murderers often went about in splendid costumes. Another parallel was offered by the book's binding; *de luxe* editions never guaranteed the quality of the content. The first pages of the praise were devoted to the idea that often the things we find annoying are in fact useful when studied in more detail. The key question was: what is really harmful to human beings? Obviously, it was something that took away men's health, wealth or life. Usually, diseases and death were placed in this category, and therefore, Czanakius also studied the concepts of disease and pain. The discussion seemed to elaborate parodically on Stoic syllogisms, which were intended to prove that pain was unpleasant, but it actually did not make life worse, and thus pain was not an evil.

First, Czanakius noted that no one was free of disease, since men always had wounds somewhere on their bodies, caused by knives, oars, ploughs or other tools that were invented to satisfy their needs and help them in the acquisition of wealth (p. 2). Wounds could strike deep; they were dangerous and also morally dubious in view of how many of them arose. However, Czanakius denied that the itch belonged to such evils and set out to demonstrate his belief by stressing the ambiguity of the term "disease" (p. 4). If disease was something that stung (*pungit*) the body, then lice, fleas, sultry weather or severe cold, which all caused a stinging feeling, were considered diseases. Or if disease was something that bit (*mordet*) the body, then all biting animals should, with good reason, be included in this class. Thus, disease was not synonymous with physical pain. If disease was defined as being against nature (*praeter naturam*), then everything taking place in unnatural ways was classified as a disease: premature baldness, grey hair on a young man's head or any stroke of luck, like a golden tripod found in the sea by fishermen (p. 5). In Czanakius's words, medical doctors distinguished good health from disease by saying that disease caused damage, first to the faculties and then to action. However, scabies did not have any such ill effects. Briefly, scabies differed from disease in that it was not pernicious to humans.

The definitions of disease employed here remind one of Cicero's definitions of pain in the second Book of his *Tusculan disputations*, as well as Seneca's discussions of grief and pain in his *Epistles* (99.14; cf. Wilson 1997, p. 56). It is also possible to discover here echoes of the views presented of disease in contemporary medical literature. In his *Institutiones medicinae*, Daniel Sennert first discussed whether disease was something natural or against nature. Then he observed that good health was defined as an ability to act (1628, p. 10), whereas disease meant a temporary inability to perform those actions and tasks that were natural to men. Sennert disapproved of the Galenic view of disease as a cessation of all actions – in that case all men who were for some reason motionless should be considered ill, be the reason for their immobility sleep, darkness or leisure. Instead, disease should be understood in terms of a momentary inability to perform one's normal and necessary actions (p. 137).[35]

Thus, Czanakius saw that the itch was in fact a healthy state par excellence, because, instead of hampering the human faculty or preventing the patient from desired activities, it drew the body's forces together, stimulated the mind and convoked all the finger- and toenails to join the scratching, even to the extent that the patient learned to despise his nightly sleep (p. 6).

In addition to finding arguments appealing to conceptual clarity and tenable definitions, Czanakius defended the itch for ethical reasons. The itch improved the moral condition by making lazy men industrious (they scratched) and by releasing new energies. Hands were kept busy, unlike at leisure. Leisure (*otium*) was to be blamed, since many diseases ensued from or were aggravated by leisure; a divine example of this error was Jupiter who in his idleness ruined his reputation by having affairs with Leda and Europa (p. 8). The itch acquired morally protective qualities and seldom attacked men who exercised daily, that is, athletes and workmen; it frequently found its target among the leisurely, soft gentlemen and especially students. The academic background of the parodic praise was evident in the reference to a common proverb that defined the student as a scabby animal who lacked money (p. 8, *Studiosum esse animal scabiosum, carens pecunia*). Interestingly, Otium was at times personified as a woman who was blind, led by a rope held by Inertia, and lacking hands, as if she never needed the means with which to do human work (Vickers 1985, p. 12). The itch, by contrast, was all about the hands; it kept men awake around the clock and abolished all tendency towards illicit inactivity. The strongest argument in favour of the itch was its ability to improve character and make the patient hardworking and active. Laziness or sloth (*pigritia*) was the primary vice cured by the itch (p. 7). Czanakius rhetorically described laziness as a sweet toxin, spiny (*spinosa*) softness, poisonous Circe, a siren song, Colchian art (referring to Medea) and an evil spirit, giving to it attributes that were the conventional images of sin and malice. Laziness called forth frivolous thoughts, disturbed thinking; it led to wars and was the reason that the last king of the Assyrian Empire, Sardanapalus, noted for his licentiousness and luxury, as well as Julius Caesar lost their realms (p. 8). In Czanakius's words, like a military commander, the itch attacked the strongest of enemies, laziness, and also directed its forces against another mighty opponent, the vice of intemperance (p. 9).

Very similar ethical arguments were made by Petrarch in his *De remediis utriusque fortunae* (II.85, *De scabie*). For example, the itch kept men active around the clock and although the disease itself was annoying, the cure was noble, consisting of hard work, diet and patience. Besides, it was always better to suffer from a visible skin-disease than from cupidity and lust, the itches of the soul (*animorum scabies, cupiditas ac libido*; cf. Augustine, *Confessiones* 9.1.1: *scabies libidinum*). Petrarch remarked that the itch taught men two important virtues, diligence and patience.

To return to Czanakius, these ethical aspects were followed by a discussion of scratching as generating both delight (*delectatio*) and pleasure (*voluptas*) rather than pain. The concept of delight was often used for uplifting and spiritual satisfaction obtained from intellectual activities, whereas pleasure resided in the senses and was felt by satisfying physical demands. For Cicero, *delectatio* was precisely the pleasure obtained through the senses (*Tusc.* 4.9.20). But here the two kinds of pleasures were interchangeable, which emphasised the overall positive effects and joys obtained from scratching. In the manner of the Epicureans (cf. Wilson 1997, p. 56), Czanakius saw pain as the polar opposite of pleasure. If pleasure was the highest good that resulted from virtue and rendered men happy, as it was with the Epicureans, then the itch was, with good reason, glorified as the source of consummate pleasure. The itch titillated the body as music tickled the mind, but the crucial difference was that music (Orfeus' song, lullabies) made men drowsy, dulled their senses, closed the eyes, stopped the ears and rendered all limbs languid (p. 11). In contrast, ticklish pustules kept the patient awake, abolished all sleepiness, awakened the senses and mobilised the body members (p. 12). This laboriousness was accompanied by the unending pleasures of titillation, but very much unlike that received in sex, where after much effort the pleasure was brief and followed by sadness, sometimes by regret (p. 11). Celsus had noted in his medical discussion of scabies that it sometimes turned to a persistent and rapidly spreading itching ulceration, and the more the itching, the more difficult it was to relieve (*De medicina* 5.28.16). But in Czanakius's opinion, if the itch caused wounds – external signs of immorality – then the disease was not to be blamed but rather the excessive scratching (pp. 6–7). A harmless itch was turned into ulcers by the patient's own restless and impudent finger nails; the patient in his excessive seeking after pleasure had abused itch and had himself caused the damage. Likewise, very healthy and useful things such as bread, honey and nectar could also cause damage when used to excess. Thus, everything in nature could be corrupted by abuse.

Aesthetic grounds were also given here to defend the colourful pustules that decorated the body and rivalled nature in beauty (pp. 13–14). Rainbows, crystals, tulips, stars, beautiful landscapes and other colourful things and treasures of nature lost out to the flaming beauty of the scabby body. Especially interesting was Czanakius's comparison between the itch and precious stones and jewels, traditionally, the epitome of vanity and luxury (pp. 14–16). These gems were found deep in the earth, whereas the itch brought the beauty to the surface, making it easily visible to all. Moreover, the itch did not just decorate fingers, which were proudly exhibited to everyone, but covered the whole body with colourful configurations, which were, however, concealed from alien eyes. Unlike jewelry, the itch did not make its bearer arrogant or evoke envy in others; neither did it require riches from its owner, but was obtained for free. Czanakius recalled the story of a rich man who was travelling across a thick forest between London and Oxford where his splendid ring attracted a group of bandits. The robbers severed the man's fingers when they were unable to remove his ring. Czanakius himself, as a poor student, had passed through the forest safely. Likewise, Juvenal had noted that a rich man carrying his treasures with him takes every stirring shadow for a sword, whereas the empty-handed traveller passes the highwaymen without worries, singing and whistling (Juvenal 10.22, *cantabit vacuus coram latrone viator*; cf. Boethius, *De consolatione philosophiae* II.5.34).

Czanakius also identified two kinds of women to illustrate the ethical superiority of the itch to rings and jewels (p. 16): "Jewels seem to me like public whores, whereas the itch is like an honest matron or a virgin. The prostitutes publicly display themselves in the squares and theatres [...], but the decent wives and bashful maidens always remain hiding at home, in the shadows of their houses and inside domestic walls." Unlike prostitutes, the itch and decent women were carefully covered by clothes. Scabies was thus paradoxically both visible and hidden. And when jewels were used against certain diseases to abolish excess fluids from the body, the itch was an even better remedy, since it cured disorders of the lazy and intemperate mind (p. 18). Therefore, it was called both pharmacy and theriac of the mind and the body (p. 21).

Yet another reason to defend scabies was related to reverence: scabby people were highly esteemed by everyone, evident in the distance kept from them (p. 17). The distance and the patient's typical isolation were here interpreted as signs of the patient's high self-esteem and the social respect shown to him. The scabby man was compared with other arrogant creatures – woman, horse and peacock – in his sense of superiority. The distance was not a signal of shame, abhorrence, disgust or fear of infection, but rather a sign of reverence. The same conclusion was also made in an anecdote in *Nugae venales* (p. 22) that asked what are the privileges of scabby people? The response was: "If three chaps are at the table and there are only two glasses, then the scabby gentleman is always afforded a glass of his own. He is also allowed to enjoy the privilege of drinking, eating and shitting alone in peace." Other benefits mentioned were that he slept alone and showed off his beautiful colours, which surpassed the glory of leprosy.

On old age

Even though fever, gout and scabies were shown in many ways to outdo other ills, other infirmities were also capable of tempering the physical appetites. For example, Cicero had famously lauded old age in his *De senectute*, giving several reasons for its superiority over youth. First, old people were not forced to withdraw from all active employment, since active study and learning ended only with death. Second, even if age reduced physical strength, the strength of the intellect remained and even grew stronger. Third, lack of sensual pleasures was a blessed thing and facilitated life, since pleasures darkened the soul. Furthermore, sensual pleasures gave way to intellectual pleasures. Thus, dignified old people remained active until the last and their old age was spent in happiness, free of the desires that troubled the young soul.

Likewise, Plutarch noted in his essay "On moral virtue" that "in old men the source of desire, which is seated about the liver, is in the process of being extinguished and becoming small and weak, whereas reason increases more and more in vigour as the passionate element fades away together with the body" (*Moralia* 450F; trans. W. C. Helmbold). The mind was thus dependent on the constitution of the body and its faculties. Old men were wise not only because of their long experience and the wisdom acquired during their lifetimes, but also because their bodies had become languid, thereby naturally reducing and taming the desires. Plutarch argued that "the emotional part springs up from the flesh as from a root and carries with it its quality and composition" ("On moral virtue", *Moralia* 451A; trans. W. C. Helmbold). Seneca congratulated himself that age had not done any damage to his mind, which now had only a slight connection with his body (*Epistulae* 26.2).

This attitude towards aging partly explains the logic of disease eulogies, too, since a weak body of necessity abstained from all indulgences. Cicero's famous treatise and its arguments were imitated and echoed by the later writers of paradoxes. His wisdom was put in verse by a Scottish physician and poet Arthur Johnston (ca. 1579–1641). In his short poem *Laus senis* (1666, p. 277), Johnston reminded his readers that although there was no medicine against old age, it brought consolation to men and liberated them from many worries. These men were wise too, proven by the fact that the Roman senate consisted of old men and that young people obeyed the advice given by their elders. War was always a threat to young men: "When called up by the trumpeter, the young were forced to join the army against the enemy, / whereas the old man could stay hiding at home. / Young men make war and feel the joy of a conquered enemy / but the old merely recollect it in their memory and help others to remember." Even certain vices were allowed older people, since no one was surprised about their stinginess, unkindness or loquacity. Johnston concluded that "if there is something to be blamed in an old man's manners, blame his years and / praise the man, since the only culprit is his age." In such satirical eulogies and paradoxes, things that were commonly regarded as harmful or useless were now praised as offering gains for the sufferer, be they pains or the physical weakness of old age.

To conclude, disease eulogies were often philosophical in the sense of being consolatory. They were written as self-consolations by authors who themselves suffered from bad health or they were dedicated to sick addressees to comfort them and to furnish strength in their malady.

In their healing words the authors argued that either the evil had no existence or that the evil was not serious. Humour was also important in satirical consolations. In his consolation to gout patients, Balde, who himself had poor health (Knepper 1904, p. 38), apologised for his playful tone but reminded of the benefits of jesting (1661, question 39). Just as in the book of Proverbs (31.7) Solomon had advised the oppressed to drink wine and forget their afflictions and misery, so Balde aspired to create a Hippocrene, a fountain of solace for the diseased, and offer the afflicted a potion seasoned with the sweet and liquid jests of the fountain of the nymph Aganippe, so that they would not constantly ruminate on their suffering. Dissociating himself from the Galenic healing method, which either killed or cured the patient, Balde chose another practice in which the sonority and playfulness of the verses worked as an antidote to pain and made life easier. When normal pharmaceuticals were insufficient, Balde claimed to have unlocked a medical bag of *eutrapelia*, meaning the social virtue of wit and jesting familiar from Aristotelian ethics.[36]

Other disease eulogies and consolations often expressed similar objectives. *Podagraegraphia*, which was also entitled "a consolatory booklet", emphasised that consolations were not to be sought in pharmacies or medical treatises, but in a book that called "philosophy the best kind of medicine", for it exhilarated and cured the mind (p. 232). Disease eulogies took the role of philosophy in consoling the afflicted, and the arguments against the grief caused by suffering were culled from ancient philosophical sources.

In the next chapter, I will examine how sensory disabilities were thought to promote moral health in satirical and paradoxical discussions and how this view had its main background in (ancient) Stoic learning, which the authors of satirical paradoxes playfully employed. The genre of consolation is also relevant in this reading. Instead of offering solace in the face of death or exile, as was the case in classical consolations, the texts studied here reminded the readers why disabilities such as blindness are not to be feared. In the following pages I will examine how – in the manner of Juvenal's thirteenth satire – consolations can be simultaneously satirical.

4
Wonderfully Unaware: Sensory Disabilities, Contemplation and Consolation

Blindness and sin

The issue of the five senses belonged to philosophical or psychological discussions already in antiquity.[1] Aristotle was known as the first influential author who explained the functions of the sense organs in his *De anima* and in *De sensu*. His influence was strong in Renaissance studies, which dealt with the human mind and defended the usefulness of the senses. In *Liber de anima* (1540), Philip Melanchthon wrote, by reference to Plato, that sight was the most valuable of the senses and it helped men to learn Divinity (p. 72). Another important context for these observations was medieval and religious ethics, which identified the senses as potential threats to men's morals, seeing the eyes as windows, gateways and passages through which not only good impulses and the doctrine of faith, but also different vices, temptations and the seven deadly sins could reach the soul (Schleusener-Eichholz 1985, pp. 884–91; Vinge 1975, pp. 47–70). Satirical disease eulogies made use of several of the commonplace images and arguments found in such works as the tenth book of Augustine's *Confessiones*, Vincent of Beauvais's *Speculum morale*, Jacopone da Todi's thirteenth-century poetry and Caelius Rhodiginus's early sixteenth-century compilation entitled *Lectiones antiquae*, all of which included discussions of the senses. The topic of perception also belonged to rhetorical exercises in which orators disputed the merits of the five senses (Claren 2003, p. xix, n. 25; Esser 1961, p. 144).

Praising eyes and seeing was a conventional topic in university orations. In his speech *De visu & caecitate oratio* delivered to new masters graduates at Tübingen in 1587, a professor of Greek and Latin, Martin Crusius (Martin Kraus, 1526–1607), eloquently praised the gift of seeing, although he admitted that a piercing inner vision was an even rarer gift. Following the Aristotelian view of the usefulness of sight, Crusius argued that the capacity for seeing had enabled Anaximander, one of the earliest philosophers of the Ionian school, to discover the equinox and the solstice; it had enabled men to create and develop sciences and had helped prophets, evangelists and apostles to learn Divinity. Sight was lauded as the most important of the five senses, its great value being evident from the eyes' location in the head, significantly situated above the rest of the body. This argument was traditional and familiar from the second Book of Cicero's *De natura deorum*. God had wisely given men two eyes instead of one, so that they would see to the right and left simultaneously and not in one direction only. The eyes' significance was also proved by their helpfulness in work and building up society, including its different fields of trade, agriculture, winegrowing, architecture and navigation. Darkness, by contrast, was a malady, as it had been in Egypt, and Crusius gave several historical examples of men dazzled by some external source, such as snow or the sun seen in eclipse. Crusius had a strong Christian emphasis in his speech, and he condemned blindness in the sense of not obeying God. According to Philip Molstetter's *Laus caecitatis* (1593), even the original sin was set in motion the moment Eve saw the forbidden fruit. A different opinion, however, was expressed in *Podagraegraphia* (p. 254), which stated that there was dispute about the reason for the Fall, with both Eve and the serpent blamed. According to Gout who is speaking here, Eve wrongly blamed the serpent for the first sin, while the serpent equally erroneously accused the delicious-looking fruit. Gout refused to find fault with the sight of the apple or with seeing it, but called for the control of reason and God's will. Moreover, the gout patient who appealed to his innocence was equally in the wrong.

Crusius assessed seeing as a useful ability that had morally elevating effects on human life, whereas blindness equalled sin and ignorance. This idea has penetrated western thinking in general, and in beliefs concerning the meaning of blindness, the metaphorical parallel between the physical and the mental (or the moral) has been widely acknowledged. Roman satires included many references to various forms and degrees of blindness and defects of visual perception with people being depicted as dazzled or completely blind. Defective vision was usually interpreted morally, and it implied spiritual blindness and false judgement, the blind men's reluctance to see themselves in a true light. In

Persius' third satire the reluctant student smeared olive oil in his eyes to irritate them and thus to avoid studying (3.44–5). In Horace's satire people smeared ointment in their eyes when examining their own faults, whereas the foibles of others were viewed with the eye of an eagle or the Epidaurian snake, this animal being famous for its sharp sight (1.3.25–7).[2] Love was often blind to the loved one's blemishes, but most often in satires the eye was fooled by the golden surface, riches and fame. In Horace's satires people were captivated by the glitter of silver and bronze, and the insane eye was dazzled by the shining tableware (1.4.28; 2.2.5). Landino noted that the word *acies* (pupil) here referred to the sharpness of the eye as well as the mind (1486, *ad loc.* 2.2).

Satires, of course, viewed outward appearances and the perceptions of them as misleading and delusory. In Horace's words, Glory dragged people in chains behind her dazzling chariot (*Sermones* 1.6.23). Glittering surfaces, golden tableware, money or fame dazzled, and gold created illusions of something good and worth reaching for, but behind the scenes the satirist found sore areas and internal ugliness. Unable to see beneath the surface, the blind man based his actions on false values, wrong conclusions and an unreal self-image, and blindness distorted his cognition of reality (cf. Horace, *Sermones* 2.3.43–4).

At times all of human life was judged in these terms. For example, in his *De eclipsi solari* (1662) Balde suggested that during the eclipse of 1654 the sun did not go through any change, whereas men's minds were darkened. In the preface to his satire *Arx virtutis sive de vera animi tranquillitate*, Johannes Havraeus (Jan van Havre, b. 1551) couched his writing in medical terms, saying that he hastened to fight against a common disease, hoping that men would learn to know themselves with the help of their sickness and pain and allow doctors to medicate their inner ulcers (1627, p. 9).[3] In his first satire Havraeus employed an image of universal blindness, praying for people to be relieved of it and have their eyes opened to realise the mindlessness of the world (*caeco velamine adempto, / perspicere his qui terrenis in sordibus haerent*). The motif of mental blindness recurred in Havraeus's first satire, identified with specific passions like desire (*caeca cupido*), luxury (*luxuries* [...] / *aut hebetans aut obcaecans caligine sensus*), love (*caeci flammas amoris*), and hunger for gold and for public honour (*caecat & urit / exsecranda fames auri, & popularis honoris*). All of these equalled blindness in the sense of losing oneself and misunderstanding the true value of things. Echoing Seneca's images of mental blindness (*Epistulae* 122.4), Havraeus stressed that he was born for something better than being merely a slave to his body (*sat.* 2). Havraeus adopted numerous expressions from

Roman satire, including pathological ulcers, guilty pallor and putrid filth swelling inside the body. In Havraeus' vision, God blinded the man he wished to destroy. In the manner of Horace, he declared that in their blind self-love, men viewed their own vices with the eye of a pigeon, but others' shortcomings, with the eye of a hawk (*sat.* 3).

In ancient tradition, blindness was often associated with guilt and punishment. The blind were burdened with culpability or a serious offence, such as having seen the gods. The intervention of gods or demons in blinding a person was understood as a punishment for the transgression of a basic natural, moral or religious law, and blindness reminded of this guilt (Barasch 2001, pp. 21–8). The ancient seer Tiresias, who became a stock figure in early modern blindness stories and gave the title to the Parisian lawyer Jacob Guther's (Jacques Gouthière or Guthierres, ca. 1575–1638) essay *Tiresias, seu caecitatis encomium* (1616) discussed below, was blinded after having seen Minerva naked. According to Guther, Minerva represented wisdom, which, once perceived, remained unforgettable. The mind was affixed to wisdom as if blind to carnal pleasures and other worldly things (pp. 270–1). According to another popular tradition (cf. Ovid, *Metamorphoses* 3.316–38), Tiresias, who had experienced life in both genders, was blinded because of his claim that women derive more pleasure from sex than do men. For this reason, Hera deprived Tiresias of sight, but Zeus gave him inner vision. Guther also mentioned the ancient Greek poet Stesichorus of Himera and the Thracian bard Thamyras as victims of similar punishments (p. 273): Stesichorus was struck blind after having blamed Helen of Troy, but he regained his sight after having composed a palinode in her favour. Thamyras was blinded when he claimed to be superior to the muses in singing. Eulogies of blindness often listed famous sightless people from ancient history and literature; these included, for example, Oedipus, the Cyclops Polyphemus and the Thracian king Polymestor, blinded by Hecuba, whose son he had slain.

Blindness and insight

In his history of the ambiguous image of blindness Moshe Barasch (2001) has noted that in ancient mythology and in western culture in general, there was another more positive idea whereby blindness was not considered evil. Even though a blind man was deprived of his most precious ability, to see and to find his way without the help of others, he was often given other gifts, such as the gift of prophecy, exceptional knowledge or an ability to communicate directly with a deity. What the blind person lost in body, he was given back in spirit and inner vision. Blindness was a dignified condition, which afflicted heroes (Oedipus) and old seers (Homer and Demodocus) and signalled spiritual insight and self-knowledge (Tiresias). Cicero had already noted that although Homer was blind, his epic appealed to the senses and conveyed all events as vividly and distinctly as if they were occurring before the audience's very eyes (*Tusc.* 5.39.114–15). Moreover, heroes like Tiresias never bemoaned their lot.

Thus, Philip Molstetter, a blind student from late sixteenth-century Mainz, wrote an encomium *Laus caecitatis*, dedicated to his patron Philip Wolff von Rosenbach, in which Molstetter sought to prove by his eloquence that he had made progress in his studies. His talk, written in poetic hexameter, recalled how he went blind in childhood and was therefore unable to see his audience, the blue sky or the green meadows. Nevertheless, he aspired to climb Mount Parnassus. In his words, before proceeding to serious studies, it was well to exercise wit through writing paradoxes. Molstetter asked his audience to hold their laughter on seeing a blind man ascend the *cathedra*, because they would learn that eloquence did not require eyes if the mind was illuminated. According to Molstetter, the seventh-century Flemish saint Audomarus went blind in old age, but when people prayed for him, he regained his sight. But soon, after having seen the corruption of the world, he begged God to blind him again, which God permitted. Thus, blindness protected men from many evils and people should in fact be congratulated for their defective vision.

Paradoxical praises inverted expectations and conventions; therefore, the capacity of seeing became morally dangerous, and blindness was represented as leading men to virtue. The authors of paradoxical disease eulogies abandoned the (Aristotelian) idea that perception could give reliable knowledge and criticised sensual pleasure. They relied on Plato, Seneca, the Church Fathers and several medieval religious writers who had regarded the sense organs as the source of wrong beliefs and potential instruments of sin. Fashionable anatomical studies and their detailed descriptions of the structure of the eye did not have much influence on Latin disease eulogies. Sensory disabilities took the role of perceptive guardians and watchmen that had earlier been attributed to the eyes; blindness protected the soul from moral evils.

Blindness was mentioned among the human miseries and adversities that could be comforted with words (Cicero, *Tusc.* 3.34.81). Consolations addressed to the blind were found, for example, in *De remediis fortuitorum*, often ascribed to Seneca who also treated blindness in some of his epistles, and Jerome's letters, which contained some examples of consolations for the blind.[4] Petrarch's *De remediis utriusque fortunae*, a store of remedies against all human miseries, is an important source text in this sense; it expanded the rhetorical remedial treatments found in earlier works. Its influence on paradoxical praises of disease has often remained unnoticed, even though George McClure, for example, observes that Petrarch's most ambitious effort as a *medicus animorum* is found in this work (1990, p. 46).[5] The second volume of Petrarch's book, written in the form of short dialogues among Reason and Dolor, deals with many illnesses which were found in paradoxical eulogies: "On Gout" (84), "On Fever" (112), "On Scabies" (85), "On Blindness" (96), "On Deafness" (97), "On Obesity" (99) and even "On Toothaches" (94). Dolor the interlocutor complains about numerous miseries, which disturb him; Reason responds with arguments that endeavour to convince him that his mourning is groundless. Even though sense perceptions are pleasant, Reason says, such pleasures are worthless and disturbing, whereas the soul of the blind man is peaceful and tranquil; happiness is found within (II.96, *De cecitate*). In addition to Petrarch, another important text in this sense was Lipsius's *De constantia*, which also emphasised the value of patience, true judgement and freedom from the emotions (such as sorrow).

According to Girolamo Cardano's *De consolatione* (1542, pp. 111–12), even though the blind had lost their animal eyes – those that they had in common with the mice and lizards – they had received the eyes of an angel – the mind's eyes that could contemplate the heavens.[6] Therefore, the blind were often exceptionally intelligent and their faculty of memory was strong. Besides, they could still enjoy many sensual pleasures. Cardano declared that being ill was very human and strengthened the mind. As Joel C. Relihan has noted when discussing Boethius's *Consolation*, all consolations include "a movement away from the physical and practical toward the ethereal and abstract"; those who are consoled are turned from their present situation towards contemplation of eternal truths (2007, p. 50). Moreover, the language of medicinal wisdom belonged to the topoi of consolation (Relihan 2007, p. 109; Morford 1973, p. 29). In his *Tusculanae disputationes* (3.34.82), Cicero noted that just as physicians treated the suffering parts of the body, so consoling words were used to heal distress (*aegritudo*). In Boethius's Menippean satire, consolation is brought by Philosophy who is extolled as medicine for the fear of death and passions of the soul, and the relation of the consoler and the consoled is presented as a doctor and his patient. Here reason is the remedy for sorrow and complaint (I.2.1, *Sed medicinae, inquit, tempus est quam querelae*).[7] The same motif of healing and a conflict between the spiritual and the secular man were found, for example, in Petrarch's *Secretum* (cf. McClure 1990, pp. 22–9), and similar argumentative structures were also used in favour of diseases.

The widely-held opinion that blindness was a misfortune was considered misleading. Guther argued that instead of relying on beliefs and opinions, one should consult ancient philosophy, which offered a different assessment of physical disabilities. Writers of paradoxes reviewed what the ancient Stoics had said on the subject and focused in more detail on the concept and nature of blindness. They asked what constituted true blindness, what blind people did not see, what they were still capable of seeing and how the disability affected their well-being. The key argument was that the disability did not deprive men from anything essential to their happiness.

Cicero, who was frequently quoted in these discussions, dealt with physical infirmities in his *Tusculanae disputationes* (5.38.110–40.117). He founded his defence of sensory disabilities on Epicurus' claim that the wise man was always happy, owing to his virtue, and thus, he was happy even in difficulties or when he was without the senses of sight or hearing. By quoting philosophers like Cicero and giving examples of happy blind men in history, the paradoxists endeavoured to change the understanding of the malady's effects on human life and to remind their readers of the supreme value of sound judgement, virtuous living and intellectual life, which blindness did not disturb. The philosophical opposition between body and mind was frequently brought out. Since the body was here a fleshly prison of the mind and secondary to it, its blindness was not as dangerous as the worse evils of mental blindness and immoral darkness, which seized wicked bodies. In the manner of ancient philosophers, the satirical authors stressed that physical diseases were without blame, but mental diseases were not.

Instead of seeing blindness as a grave physical injury to the body's essential functions, paradoxical and satirical eulogies endeavoured to prove its positive impact on human life with the example of the ancient philosophers who had deliberately deprived themselves of sight. Aulus Gellius noted in *Noctes Atticae* (10.17) that Democritus let the rays of the sun destroy his eyes in order to make his thinking and meditation more vivid and to free himself from seeing the good luck of bad citizens and other injustices in the world. As remembered, such events also stimulated satirical indignation. Although Democritus did not distinguish between black and white, he did make a clear difference between good and bad, just and unjust, honest and base, and thus had piercing moral vision. Democritus' example of voluntary blindness was mentioned in the defences of blindness by Molstetter, Guther, Vulteius, Passerat and Puteanus.[8]

At times philosophers also manipulated other body parts to sharpen their mental vision: the Academic philosopher Carneades purged his stomach with hellebore to prevent corrupt humours from rising to his mind and thereby weakening his thinking (Gellius, *Noctes Atticae* 17.15). Chrysippus used hellebore three times to clear his brain (Petronius, *Satyricon* 88). However, in this case there was nothing paradoxical in the treatment, since it was widely assumed that indigestion and heavy meals were bad for the intellect. Nevertheless, all these stories stressed that physical and mental conditions were interdependent and things that one could affect and change. In his *Satyricon* (1605, Ch. 6), John Barclay described how a virtuous man, Euphormio, pretended madness in order to conform to the European world, but tired of this pretence, took a remedy and seemed to recover from his lunacy. In addition to the overt criticism of the early seventeenth-century Europe, the passage can be read as a parodic variation of the earlier satirical cures, which sought to restore man's tranquillity and sanity.

Guther, Passerat and Puteanus on blindness

One early modern eulogy of blindness that drew upon many earlier commonplaces was written by early seventeenth-century French humanist and lawyer Jacob Guther. His *Tiresias, seu caecitatis encomium* (also known as *Tiresias, seu de caecitatis et sapientiae cognatione*) was included in two collections of playful eulogies, *Admiranda rerum admirabilium encomia* and *Dissertationum ludicrarum et amoenitatum scriptores varii*.[9] Guther first noted that the eyes had many positive effects on human life. The perception of beauty, the sun, the moon, the sky and the earth delighted man's heart, gave him considerable pleasure and passed on knowledge of eternal things (1666, p. 258). Guther quoted the saying of early Ionian philosopher Anaxagoras that men were born for a very simple reason, to see the sun. Guther reminded his readers that other ancient philosophers had also acknowledged the advantages of seeing: the Stoics claimed that thanks to the eyes, a man was closer to the gods; Aristotle argued that all the arts were invented with the help of sight; and many philosophers agreed that knowledge of the intellect depended on sense perceptions (p. 259). Eyes were useful in social life, since they expressed moral character and emotions. A single look could reveal an inner feeling of love and express modesty. Moreover, the eyes bespoke different passions: they could be unfriendly, gloomy, flaming, serious, humble, lively or dull. Eyes that swivel in an irregular manner, as if blown by the wind, were symptomatic of madness. Doctors were able to anticipate an approaching death by looking at a patient's eyes, and an inner fire burning in them was often the first signal of the onset of an acute and grave illness (p. 260).

However, Guther maintained that eyes did not feel any delight themselves, and the mind had many reasons to rejoice without the use of sight. He argued that seeing eyes were worthless unless supported and guided by a sharp intellect. Proverbially, Guther noted that often men did not see, even with their eyes open (p. 250). The argument echoed Cicero's *Tusculanae disputationes* (1.20.46) in which he observed that, though eyes and ears were open and uninjured, people did not see or hear unless the mind was active and attentive; the body alone did not have perceptions unless the soul received the objects seen. Cicero argued here against Lucretius, who had maintained that when people die the soul no longer feels or perceives (Vinge 1975, pp. 29–34). In contrast, Cicero saw that the soul could function independently of the senses. In his *De remediis* Petrarch also pointed out that the mind, not the senses, is the source of true knowledge (II.96). Guther used these earlier arguments to console the blind and together with Cicero he stressed that the wise man did not need the use of his eyes, but rather took pleasure in thinking. Likewise, Guther, referring to Epicurus, added that eyes and ears were not meant for mere sensory perception. Whereas the other three senses served the body, sight and hearing were philosophical senses that served the mind and commanded the other senses (p. 250). The ability to see with the mind's eye was a requisite for humanity. Balde compared the mind's eye with the sun, which illuminates the blind man's world from east to west and carries him from pole to pole (*Lyricorum libri* 4.20).

Guther stated that light as such did not guarantee sharpness of vision and could even cause damage: Xenophon's soldiers lost their sight when wandering around snowy countryside; in Sicily prisoners were blinded when taken from an underground cell into the light; and no one could look straight into the sun without damaging the eyes (pp. 268–9). Another commonplace, mentioned by Molstetter in his *Laus caecitatis*, was to point out that no one felt sorry if he did not see at night – how, then, could darkness be a bad thing? This remark too echoed Cicero, who had observed that night did not put an end to a happy life. By quoting Cicero (*Tusc.* 5.38.112), Molstetter also mentioned the blind Cyrenaic Antipater, whose ironic response to women who pitied him was, "Is there no pleasure in the night?"

Guther agreed with other authorities that mental blindness was a far more serious condition than mere physical blindness, which was often compensated for with virtue. Mental blindness and lack of prudence were the worst of maladies, which nothing could alleviate or cure. Guther singled out ancient blind people who were also blind mentally (p. 248). For example, Harpaste, the misshapen female clown to Seneca's wife did not recognise her own blindness, but merely asked for a guide to help exchange her quarters for a well-lit place, since her apartment felt too dark. Seneca had mentioned her in the same way: to show how few people recognise their own handicaps (*Epistulae* 50.2–4). Here Seneca also memorably observed that the evil that afflicts men is not external, but, like blindness, is situated in men's very vitals. Thus, it was difficult to attain soundness when one did not even notice the disease.

Guther continued the list with Catullus Messalinus who was blind both physically and mentally and unable to feel fear, shame or pity (cf. Juvenal 4.113). Polyphemus the Cyclops was another rough character, and, in Guther's words, his blindness was in his refusal to worship the gods or acknowledge their existence. Polyphemus denied the gods' superiority and was not afraid of them, since as a Cyclops he relied on his own strength alone – an error that especially the Christian authors repeatedly condemned, claiming that ultimately everything in men's lives was in the hands of God. Guther quoted Cicero (*Tusc.* 5.39.115) as saying that Polyphemus had no more wisdom than the rams in his herd. In his satirical pessimism, Guther added that his contemporary figures even far exceeded the old warning examples (p. 249). The phrase "of the Cyclops' sleep" also became proverbial, denoting deep and death-like slumber caused by heavy drinking (Rigault 1684). For his part, Molstetter in his *Laus caecitatis*, when looking for the essence of humanity compared visually-endowed men with animals: even though a small ant, a tiny fly, a heavy ox and a slow ass were all capable of seeing, this did not make them or anyone else human.

After having emphasised the importance of mental vision, Guther concentrated on deceptive perceptions that misguided men unless the mind showed them the right way (p. 251). The mentally blind were compared to a patient in whose liver bile abounded, producing delusions and hallucinations. Perturbations and diseases of the mind made man believe in his false visions. Likewise, someone who received a blow to his eye saw everything in red; to a choleric patient, everything seemed yellow. False visions were illusions, in Greek *phantasiai*, which had nothing truthful in them. Mentally blind fools who combated reason were compared to *andabatae*, the type of Roman gladiators who fought wearing helmets without eyeholes. *Andabatae* was also the name of one of Varro's Menippean satires. Distorting mirrors were mentioned as a yet another typical mine of misinformation, which made an object seem smaller or larger than it actually was and turned it upside down so that man's feet were unnaturally above his head or caused confusion between the right and left sides (p. 252).[10] In such reflected images the external objects existed, but since they were perceived incorrectly, they could deceive. Irrational desires also affected perception. Guther recalled the famous Aesopian fable of a greedy dog which, seeing the reflection of the meat it was carrying in a pool of water, tried to snatch at it but dropped the meat, losing it forever to the water (p. 269).

Such reflections illustrated the diseased condition of the soul. The sick soul based its activities on false visions and misjudgements, owing to the impact of passions on the perceptions and (through them) on the rational faculty. The wise man was able to control his appetites, but certain passions such as cupidity – described by Cicero as a "blind and thoughtless mistress of the soul" (*De inventione* 1.2.2) – tended to take hold of men's actions. In Guther's words, the desires of ambition and love were given the adjective "blind" and compared with eternal sleep, which impeded rational decision-making (pp. 252–4). Cupid or Eros was frequently depicted blindfolded, reflecting the blindness of the emotion. Guther substantiated these commonplaces by references, for example, to Menander's comedies ("to advise a lover to obey wisdom was a wasted effort"). In his *Laus caecitatis*, Molstetter noted how one single look bound sad Dido's heart to Aeneas and how her mind burned at the sight of the beloved. Molstetter concluded that this inner fire was impossible to smother and finally resulted in Dido's suicide, significantly, by self-immolation. In his *De eclipsi solari* (1662), Balde added that had Dido been blind or even one-eyed she would have survived (poem 3).

Fortuna, another personification of an abstract idea, was also famous for appearing blindfolded, symbolising that luck was always changing and had no rational grounds but distributed welfare at random (Barasch 2001, p. 123; Schleusener-Eichholz 1985, p. 567). In Hutten's dialogue *Fortuna* (1519), the goddess was blinded by Jupiter, because with vision she would have delivered her gifts to the good and the deserving, which in Jupiter's reasoning would only make them effeminate and corrupt them (1860, p. 79). In Guther's encomium, Fortuna was both insane and blind, but by appealing to the Stoics, Guther stressed that fortune did not determine whether one lived a good or a bad life, because she only affected the circumstances over which a wise man was able to rise and thereby show himself stronger than the gifts or the miseries such as blindness bestowed by Dame Fortuna (p. 255). Avarice was also mentioned as a vice that turned men blind. This vice, represented here in the figure of Plutus, a god of wealth, was in Guther's view especially dangerous in leaders and readily led men into war (pp. 255–6). In Aristophanes' play *Plutus* this god was a sickly old man whom Zeus had blinded so that he could not tell the good from the undeserving. Therefore the gifts of money were distributed unevenly in human society, and there was no correlation between possessions and merit. The personified Poverty claimed that she was the source of every blessing in men's lives, since she compelled men to earn their daily bread, disciplined them and made them hardworking.[11]

In addition to Cupid, Fortuna and Plutus, the fourth blindfolded god mentioned by Guther was Iustitia (pp. 256–7), whom the ancient Egyptians had imagined as being headless. The most plausible explanation given here for Iustitia's blindness was that her will was led by the sight of her reason and took illumination from its light, just as the blind were led by a full-sighted guide. Reason was here ennobled above the senses, and moral conflicts experienced by man were represented as clashes between reason and the senses.

Satirical paradoxes emphasised the importance of moral seeing, and the difficulty of distinguishing between vice and virtue was repeatedly used as an argument for blindness. Guther argued that the riches of the world, the pursuit of honours and of physical delights were falsely regarded as valuable by people who thought that they could find happiness in pleasures or in the gifts of Fortuna (p. 263). He illustrated such blindness by the blind man who fell into a pit, a humorous figure familiar from ancient anecdotes and fables, but here the falling man did not stand for an intellectual absorbed in cerebration and hence, was absent-minded; instead, he represented a man whose path was guided by his passions instead of his reason (p. 253). The main argument in favour of blindness remained that the bad influences and dangers that disturbed the balance of the mind came from outside the body and reached men through the senses. Seeing the object increased the desire to seize it. Guther used Pliny's *Naturalis historia* as a source for unusual cases, such as the story of the Illyrians who killed each other with their evil eyes, this being given as an extreme and a concrete reminder of the fact that blindness protected men from bad influences (p. 261).

With reference to another old commonplace, Guther claimed that physical blindness was compensated for by virtue and a deeper sense of seeing, governed by wisdom. This idea was once again proved with a list of ancient, virtuous blind men that owed most of its names to Cicero (*Tusc.* 5.38.112–39.115). These included Appius Claudius Caecus, who in Cicero's words was blind for many years, yet performed his public and private duties impeccably. According to Guther, Appius saw more clearly than the senators that peace with Pyrrhus would result in slavery (p. 262). Molstetter, Vulteius and Puteanus all included Appius among the virtuous blind men who persuaded his citizens to turn down Pyrrhus' peace proposals.

Among ancient blind men, Cicero and Guther also singled out philosophers like Democritus, and other sightless wise men, such as Gnaeus Aufidius and a Roman grammarian Quintus Asconius Pedianus, both of whom wrote histories without being able to see (p. 265). Using the device of *praeteritio* and directing the attention to that which he refrained from saying, Guther mentioned a courageous hero, Timoleon of Corinth, who became blind a short time before his death in 337 BC. Demetrius blinded himself in order to penetrate nature's secrets; an Epicurean philosopher Metrodorus pierced his eyes so that they would not disturb his contemplation (p. 267). Guther's consistent argument was that a wise man did not need eyes, and his vision was sharper without them. If one eye was damaged, the other grew stronger. Taken to its logical conclusion, if both eyes were missing, the mind became even more perceptive. Petrarch also mentioned many of these ancient men in his praise of blindness (*De remediis* II.96). And according to Molstetter, becoming virtuous resembled growing old, since the old are naturally blind but are also wise and virtuous.

Among his contemporaries, Guther made reference to French satirist and poet Jean Passerat (1534–1602), who towards the end of his life had become blind and, in order to console himself, had delivered a public speech *De caecitate* (Lyon, 1597) in defence of blindness. Passerat emphasised his blindness in the latter part of his speech by repeating several times *caecus sum*, yet each time denying this to be a bad condition. Passerat's *De caecitate*, also included in Dornau's *Amphitheatrum* (pp. 262–4), listed the conventional examples of blindness (love, Plutus, Fortuna, Democritus, Tiresias, Oedipus, Appius, famous singers and poets like Stesichorus, Thamyras, Antipater). Following tradition, Passerat argued that seeing made men prone to many vices and evoked such disturbing emotions as love, hate, joy, sadness, fear and desire, which caused glaucoma in the intellect. Men were forced to see painful things they abhorred – acts of adultery, incest and nocturnal ghosts – whereas blindness – synonymous with innocence – protected them from sorrows.[12] Passerat backed up his point by references to Plautus' descriptions of blind anger in *Amphitryo* and *Asinaria*. The speech also contained many references to Virgil's *Aeneid* and *Georgica*, Ovid's *Metamorphoses* and Lucretius' *De rerum natura* in illuminating different aspects of blindness, the horrors of seeing and the dark underworld.

Several comparisons were used to give perspective to blindness; in belittling the troubles it caused, Passerat likened blindness to sleep and to the deeper, metaphorical darkness of human life. The distinction between seeing and not-seeing was blurred by reminding one of the omnipresence of blindness and its different degrees and forms, such as absentmindedness and failing to notice what was close at hand. Passerat's speech closed with a reminder of the moral benefits afforded by blindness. It taught men modesty and industriousness; even judges benefited from blindness when learning to enquire into things more deeply and in understanding that the real causes behind events may not be obvious or easily perceived.

The popularity of the topic was also evident in Belgium, where the humanist Erycius Puteanus (1574–1646) published his essay *Caecitatis consolatio* in 1609. It was written to be a solace in suffering – not as an antidote to the disease – and to comfort his friend, politician and jurist Willem Criep (1535–1610), whose sight had deteriorated during his last years (De Landtsheer 2000, p. 210). Puteanus's text has been described as a philosophical treatise with a strong affinity to Stoa (De Landtsheer 2000, p. 228), but it also easily fits the loose category of paradoxical encomia with at least occasional ironic tones. Puteanus's main arguments for blindness were similar to those of others. True blindness was not physical but was defined as the mind captured by vain, incidental and external things (p. 17). Puteanus observed that even though the blind were deprived of certain pleasures of seeing, there were other means of enjoyment and of perceiving: the sun's warmth could be enjoyed without seeing; the sky, contemplated by the mind's eye, and the earth touched (p. 18). Blindness was divine, since it enveloped a man like the clouds and mist created by the gods to conceal the epic heroes, Ulysses and Aeneas (p. 19). Blindness protected man from evil and gave him freedom and peace to move unnoticed in the world in the manner of these ancient heroes. Whole families owed their surnames to their lack of sight – Caeci, Caecilii, Orbilii, Scipiones (p. 20).[13] Puteanus also gave the conventional list of blind poets, including Homer, Tiresias, Stesichorus, Thamyras and Demodocus, and philosophers, like Democritus, Diodotus,[14] the Peripatetic philosopher Xenarchus and Didymus Alexandrinus (pp. 64–6). According to Johannes Ravisius Textor's (1480–1524) similar list of blind men, Diodorus and Didymus were noted experts in geometry, even though they needed help in drawing geometrical figures.[15] Of contemporaries Puteanus mentioned his friend and professor of Latin in Perugia, Marcus Antonius Bonciarius, whose body was deformed – Puteanus perhaps exaggerated when he said that there was no discernible human feature in his figure – but since his tongue and mind were unharmed, Bonciarius was the embodiment of learning.

Puteanus relied on the topos that physical infirmities were always less harmful than those of the mind and argued that most seeing people were blind to truth and virtue. Eyes were the weakest part of the body – fragile, easily injured and thus signalling overall physical weakness (pp. 30–1). Quoting passages from Seneca's *Consolatio ad Marciam* and epistles, Puteanus argued that metaphorically, all men lived in darkness if they heeded their passions and false affections (pp. 22–3).[16]

But the concepts of blindness and darkness were studied further in order to show that both were more positive than usually credited. Darkness and night not only offered a refuge for idlers, but also the thick, unbroken shadows implied the presence of a deity, as Seneca had remarked in his epistle (41.3) and Tacitus, in his *Germania*. Far from being dangerous, the shadows were the poets' loci for creation and inspiration (pp. 25–6). Thus, the blind man found the sacred grove of the Muses, Helicon and Parnassus in his very infirmity. Here, Puteanus paradoxically connected darkness with the idea of poetical creation and the mind's work, which was more often associated with piercing light. But the blind man became an eye for himself, illuminating his world with his own intellect and the fire that kindled in his breast, without needing either a torch or direct sunlight (p. 35). In these arguments Puteanus frequently relied on Seneca's letters and the fifth book of Cicero's *Tusculanae disputationes*.

As in all defences of blindness, Puteanus also attributed many advantages to the disability. For example, blindness promoted affection among family members and fostered individual freedom. Loved ones became dear to the blind when their company was continually needed, and the wife's affection grew deeper on helping her husband (p. 27). The blind man was released from the domination of the calendar and the clock; he could freely pursue his own schedule regardless of the man-made hours or the timing of the sun and wake up when he wished (p. 28). Other senses became stronger when they took over the tasks of the eyes; the blind man learned by touching (p. 39). One of the most important benefits was that blindness allowed the contemplation of God, who was not approached by seeing or hearing but only by thinking, since only the mind could truly see and hear (p. 60, with quotations from Cicero and Plutarch's *De sollertia animalium: Mens vidit, mens audit: reliqua omnia, caeca & surda*). Blindness itself did not deprive anyone of true pleasures, which were of the mind; it was useless to cover the bedroom walls with mirrors in expectation of erotic scenes (p. 38). This may contain a reference to Seneca's *Quaestiones naturales* (1.16), which described similar mirror images, and potentially to Suetonius' *Life of Horace*, which told how the poet lined his bedroom with mirrors, in order to see erotic acts from every angle. Moreover, by protecting the mind from desires and calamities, blindness favoured tranquillity and improvement of the mind (p. 40). Seeing such things as adultery, others' successes or beautiful women seduced men just as flying insects were drawn to a flame, which then burned them to death; vices merely became stronger when warmed by vision (p. 52). Seeing resulted in unhappiness by filling men with futile desires; by inducing them to immoral actions, it also gradually produced evil characters. Among the vices caused by seeing, were, according to Puteanus, sexual desire, jealousy, envy, avarice, luxury and cruelty (pp. 44–6, 51). In contrast, blindness protected virtue, made happiness possible and was defined as innocent (p. 52). Puteanus repeatedly backed up these points by quoting Cicero's epistles and Quintilian's declamations.[17]

In contemporary medical literature blindness and sense perceptions were usually discussed without moral implications. For example, in his *Institutiones medicinae* Daniel Sennert described different false visions, wherein white things were perceived as yellow or men experienced double visions (1628, p. 308). He also noted that the glaucoma-affected eye was veiled as if with clouds or fumes (p. 386). However, these were caused by diseases and functional defects in the eye and did not imply any moral failure or suggest the patient's ignorance.

In seventeenth-century philosophy the relationship between knowledge and the senses was subject to renewed inquiries. Philosophers asked whether sound knowledge was dependent on the senses or whether it was formed in the mind. Early modern scholars also wondered why the mind was deceived by the senses. Sennert dealt with sense perceptions in the seventh Book of his *Epitome naturalis scientiae* and argued that there were two kinds of qualities, material objects and their images (such as the colours); these were by no means suspicious or deceptive (1633, p. 556ff.). He also emphasised the mind's active role in perception. Descartes was sceptical about sense perceptions and assumed that such qualities as colours, sounds and tastes were impressions caused by corporeal movements on the sense organs and their perception depended on the disposition of the soul. Likewise, Hobbes warned not to attribute the qualities perceived to the objects. Instead, knowledge depends on interior images, which men formed in their minds. (Vinge 1975, pp. 135–6.)

By taking up the subject of perception, paradoxical eulogies reflected contemporary medical and philosophical discussions. However, in disease eulogies sense perceptions were always connected with immorality, as they had been in the medieval tradition. Sounds and visions were temptations of the outer world, perceived by an individual, and problematic for many reasons. First, they were produced by the mechanical and materialistic world that satirists and a number of (Platonic) philosophers regarded as inferior to a real and true experience.[18] Therefore, the authors of paradoxes belittled the harm resulting from unseen material and unimportant objects, such as the bed one slept in or the food one ate (Puteanus 1609, p. 26). Second, sense perceptions themselves could be interpreted as unreal in that they lacked substance and were mere illusions and appearances, these being the main targets of any satirical attack. Being mere tricks and reflections, they were potentially deceptive and could lead to false judgements. Their effects were often disturbing, misleading and perplexing. These effects gained strength from men's desires and the emotions that clouded their minds. The defenders of blindness questioned the reliability of a visual experience, since it did not necessarily enable a distinction to be drawn between true and false or good and bad.

Consequently, being blind did not mean an impoverished life, since meaningful experiences were not dependent on eyesight. Satirists in general argued that most things people regarded as worth pursuing were in fact worthless, mere deceptions caused by desires that harmfully aroused the senses. Therefore, seeing material objects was insignificant or even dangerous and blindness was not an evil. For the same reason, light, rainbows, the sunrise, colours, mirror images, appearances and *fata morgana*, which were seen but did not tangibly exist, symbolised in these texts skewed human perception and the vanity of all worldly things. In contrast, by allowing men to concentrate on introspection and contemplation, blindness helped men to bypass and transcend the mortal world and became a precondition for wisdom and true knowledge. In the texts studied, consolation co-existed with a satirical reprimand against people's blindness for the misleading appearance of the world. These arguments in favour of blindness were not primarily religious, as they had been in the Middle Ages; instead, the authors relied on ancient philosophy. Moreover, eulogies of blindness were now considered paradoxical and amusing. One expression of this changing reception was seen in the inclusion of such eulogies in the large seventeenth-century anthologies of ironic encomia.

Marten Schoock on deafness

In Persius' first satire the words referring to ears (*aures* or *auriculae*) appeared several times, the diminutive being emphatically contemptuous.[19] Thirsty or hungry ears implied that men were too easily flattered and falsely relied on mellifluous words and popular opinion, apparently also in contrast to the satirist's unflattering and biting words that nonetheless conveyed truth (Persius 4.50; 2.30). Flattery was dangerous in sustaining a wrong self-image. In the same author's first satire (1.59), ears were also white. This colour can be interpreted as further emphasis on foolishness, since the whiteness of the ears referred to asses and their supposed stupidity and to the famous myth of King Midas who was given the white ears of an ass for his poor judgement and bad taste in preferring Pan's barbaric song to Apollo's (Ovid, *Metamorphoses* 11.176, *villisque albentibus*).[20] Softness of the ears had equal moral connotations, suggesting the susceptibility to flattery and overall negative weakness (Horace, *Sermones* 2.5.32–3, *molles auriculae*). The climax of Persius' first poem suggested that all human beings had asses' ears (1.121), that is to say, were foolish.[21] That man should never have stooped to the level of a beast but conquered his lower nature by reason was one of the commonplaces in all satire. Satire's common hostility towards public opinion and the masses is also discernible in these images.

Early modern authors continued these discussions about the properties of ears when considering what was proper to human beings. Georg Franck von Franckenau (1644–1704), a physician and professor of medicine at Heidelberg, supervised a dissertation on the mobile human ears, *De auribus humanis mobilibus* (1676), which belongs to his collections of texts entitled *Satyrae medicae*.[22] With references to Aristotle's *Historia animalium* (1.11), Pliny's *Naturalis historia* (11.50.136, *aures homini tantum immobiles*) and Augustine's *De civitate Dei* (14.24), for example, he argued that man is the only animal with immobile ears. Animal ears were usually larger than humans' and moved around to catch sounds, whereas human beings with small auricles had lost this ability. Since human ears were not only meant to catch inarticulate voices but also to hear articulated speech consisting of letters and syllables, it was necessary for the ears to be as stable and firm as possible. However, since the mobility of the ears was interpreted to signify deceitfulness and corruptibility and to imply that the man agreed to do anything as long as he was applauded, human ears were also here compared with an ass's ears, which differed in terms of mobility but shared a metaphorical likeness. The dissertation ended in Persius' saying that we all have the ears of an ass. Although Franck's text was primarily a medical dissertation and he also relied on such anatomical investigations as Volcher Coiter's (1534–c. 1590) *De auditus instrumento* (1572), the dissertation was clearly playful in tone. Instead of merely describing the physiology of the ear, Franck satirically employed the image of ears in a moral sense.

Writers of satirical paradoxes also invested sounds with moral meanings. Not only were sense perceptions fleeting, but they could also be dangerous, since the soul was corrupted by communication. Satires that spoke for the essential goodness of solitary life and seclusion from the world also argued that distance to possibly dangerous objects and the mortal world that had caused the sounds should be maintained, and thereby satires emphasised the uselessness of the physical senses. Sounds, frequently considered siren songs, were to be ignored without being listened to, since many errors arose not only from the things themselves, but also from the dissemination of what people said.

Once again the sources of this discussion can be traced to ancient philosophy and its ideas about the value of the senses and sense perceptions. The Stoics advised that people should transcend the mortal world altogether, whereas Cicero discussed deafness in his *Tusculanae disputationes* (5.40.116), asking if there was any real evil in it. As a harmless analogy of deafness, he mentioned the incomprehensibility of foreign languages. In Cicero's view, physical deafness was equally harmless, and deaf people were in many ways luckier than others. They avoided hearing unpleasant sounds, like thunder, the screech of a saw or the roaring sea, and reading verses was more pleasant than hearing them read aloud. In his essay "Superstition" Plutarch, for his part, remarked that tigers were provoked by the sound of beating drums, and deafness helped men attain a useful feeling of indifference and insensibility (*Moralia* 167C). Thus, sensory disabilities could actually help keep a healthy distance from the world and thereby free the mind to contemplate truth.

These philosophers' and Roman satirists' words were reflected in a 25-page essay entitled *Surditatis encomium*, written by Marten Schoock (1614–67) from Utrecht, a professor of logic at Groningen since 1640, and a notorious opponent of Descartes, whom Schoock once accused of atheism. The text was included in the *Admiranda rerum admirabilium encomia* (1666). The text defending deafness was a paradoxical encomium that also imitated earlier defences of blindness; the topic of deafness was never equally popular. For example, Johannes Ravisius Textor, who in his *Officina* gave a long list of the blind, did not offer a similar list of the deaf. However, Christian authors such as Lactantius attributed to the ear an exclusive position among the senses, since it enabled men to hear the divine word (Vinge 1975, p. 36). Augustine dealt with hearing and deafness in his ethical discussions of sense perceptions (*Confessiones* 10.33). Petrarch's *De remediis* contained a short dialogue, *De auditu perdito* (II.97), among Reason and Dolor; the latter complained about his deafness, whereas Reason assured him that deafness was useful in many ways; it protected men from flattery and other similar vices. Petrarch also noted that compared with blindness, which aroused the feelings of pity and sadness, deafness was somehow ridiculous and the deaf were often considered slightly foolish. Therefore, they were often treated with laughter.

Deafness had been previously extolled by some poets, such as Joachim Du Bellay in his "Hymne de la Surdité" (1558) and Agnolo Bronzino who had attacked the noise of church bells (Tomarken 1990, pp. 182–7). Jacob Balde's last work, *Urania victrix* (1663), contains verse epistles exchanged between Urania who represents the Christian soul and the five senses who appear as human beings. For example, a painter represents sight; a musician, hearing; a pharmacist, smell; a cook, taste, and a public-house keeper, touch. In the second book of the poem, devoted to hearing, the personified Hearing, a musician and a poet together try to persuade the soul of the usefulness of hearing, whereas Urania – the Christian soul – sarcastically refutes their arguments by demonstrating numerous advantages of deafness. Showing the senses as personifications was a medieval method and resembled, for example, Jacopone da Todi's similar allegories (Vinge 1975, p. 59).

In the manner of these texts, Schoock's discussion showed how deliberate or forced non-hearing was beneficial to an individual's moral health and not a source of misfortune. In his preface Schoock placed his text in the tradition of paradoxical praises by observing that while people have long suffered from trembling fever, knotty gout, deplorable deafness or dark blindness, they have also praised these maladies. Ears and auricles were particularly suitable objects for paradoxical praises in being small and seemingly unimportant body parts that had, however, an essential function in constituting an entrance to the mind and forming the human character.

To prepare the ground for his defence, Schoock first dealt with hearing as an indispensable ability, which made learning possible and served religion and civilisation (1666, p. 603). Hearing advanced the character, for whenever instruction and wisdom were heard, they made deep impressions on the mind, reshaped it and transformed the hearer. Ears were compared to doorways, which could be closed to harmful voices and opened to allow access to wisdom (p. 616). This image was very traditional. The medieval tradition had emphasised that faith was delivered through the ears, whereas Renaissance humanists, such as Melanchthon in his *Liber de anima* (1540), observed the usefulness of the ears in learning; he also described the anatomical structure of the ear (1846, pp. 73–4). For Schoock, hearing was also pleasurable: people took pleasure in the artful modulations of guitarists and knowingly recognised different notes and tones in their sweet music (p. 605). Speakers' skilful expressions entered the mind through the ears and their agreeable sounds caressed the sense. Regarding the crucial role of the ears in education, Persius and some early modern anecdotalists had drawn attention to the ears' cleanliness. For example, in *Nugae venales* (pp. 9–10) a short prescription studied how phlegmatic characters and those suffering from pulmonary diseases could be helped with a medicament that the author had found the previous day in a book printed thirty years before the creation: an efficient injection into the patient's ear to purge the brain of slimy and bilious humours.

Although Schoock began with the idea of hearing as a positive notion, he gradually came to have more negative thoughts about it. The sense of hearing was dangerous and capable of leading man morally astray whenever temptations, lies and desires reached the mind through the ears. Words were never mere words, but insinuated bad thoughts into men's minds and lured them to immoral actions. Lovers' deceitful words misguided or incited men to sin (p. 606). Schoock quoted Seneca's letter (31.2) on the siren song and titillating sensual pleasures in which Seneca had advised Lucilius to stop up his ears if he wished to be a wise man (pp. 615–16). It was not enough to close the ears with wax like Ulysses had made his crew to do in the *Odyssey* (12.173ff.).[23] An even denser stopper was needed, since in the present world, alluring voices did not come from one island only, but from every side.

In his epistle (56.1–2), Seneca also expressed annoyance with diverse unpleasant voices that made him hate his power of hearing. The specific context of the unpleasant uproar was the baths, a place for social gatherings in ancient times and clearly unsuitable for contemplation. In the baths the chief causes of irritation were the grunts, pants and imprisoned breaths released by the men when they exercised and the splashes of water when they swam in the pool. In the manner of Juvenal

(1.12–13) and Petronius (*Satyricon* 73), Seneca paid attention to the horrible acoustical echoes of singing and other loud voices in the bathing area from self-satisfied enthusiasts. The medley of meaningless voices also included the shrill voices of hair-pluckers, cake-sellers and sausage men advertising their products and services. Seneca argued that noises made by passing carriages, for example, filled the ears in daily life, but they were easier to ignore than human voices, which demanded attention (56.4). But Seneca insisted that no noise or uproar could upset the sound mind's thinking if it was guarded by resignation (83.7). In his *Arx virtutis*, Havraeus, when speaking for the tranquillity of the mind, also described the mindless roaring, howling and bellowing heard in the forum, and people's mad haste as if the world was on fire (1627, *sat.* 1).

Even though Schoock did not quote this specific Senecan passage, it was resonating in his criticism of hearing. In the manner of Seneca, Schoock maintained that although it was regrettable that the deaf were deprived of hearing bird song or were unable to distinguish a cuckoo from a nightingale, the loss also spared them from painful experiences and protected them from harm. Thus, deafness was no evil. Schoock singled out displeasing sounds that deaf people were spared, including verbal quarrels, the Phrygian melodies which caused insanity and the disturbing sounds of various animals – braying asses, grunting pigs, howling wolves and barking dogs (p. 607). Petrarch mentioned similar unpleasant and dangerous sounds in his *De remediis* (II.97). The deaf were safe from the furious speeches delivered by all kinds of noisy Stentores and tyrants of Morbonia, from the vehement orations delivered by the Roman orator and consul Gaius Fimbria, and from the words of Anaxagoras who taught Pericles to howl in time with the clepsydra (pp. 607–8).[24] As harmful words, Schoock also mentioned flattery and other forms of verbal deceit, referring here to Seneca who, when cautioning Lucilius against the flatterers, called them the most pernicious kind of people (p. 615).[25] Examples were taken from ancient history: the history of Rome would have been less bloody had Emperors Tiberius and Nero avoided hearing their intriguing advisers (p. 617).

Women's voices formed here a distinctive group of displeasing sounds. In satirical literature in general, female voices were often described as annoying and unpleasant (Rée 1999, p. 92). In Ben Jonson's *Epicoene, or, the Silent Woman*, for example, a gentleman had refused to take wife because he hated noise. When he finally managed to find a quiet woman and married her, she turned out to be a raucous boy. In Anatole France's *The Man Who Married a Dumb Wife*, the speechless wife's tongue was surgically removed, but to her husband's great shock, after the operation she turned into a true chatterbox. Another intervention was now needed for the husband, so his doctor made him deaf to save him from the wife's talkativeness.

Schoock's invective against female garrulity was written along similar lines. A deaf man was happily immune to painfully talkative women, whose tongues jingled like the famous wind harp of Dodona – which was quiet at least on calm days. And when the other parts of the female body fell ill, the throat was never hoarse and the tongue never suffered from ulceration. All body parts were curable when ill except the female tongue, unless it was cut off by a knife (pp. 608–9). Schoock compared female talkativeness and male quietude with animal communication and noticed that in contrast, even among the grasshoppers, the male sang loudly while the female only murmured quietly. Schoock also quoted the words of the famous Arragonian king Alphonsus, saying that marriage was happy only when the husband was deaf and the wife blind. Schoock further relied on Semonides' misogynistic passage and called the wife her husband's shipwreck, domestic storm, obstacle to silence, lifelong captivity, daily punishment, expensive battle, adorned dog and necessary evil (pp. 609–10).

Several moral and religious arguments were used to praise deafness. Unable to hear slander, deaf people did not learn malice. Nor did they learn affectation. Schoock recalled hermits and desert saints as exemplary men who had retreated to secret places (pp. 622–4). They had deliberately sought quiet in secluded caves or retreated to thick forests, fled to the open desert or to remote mountains in order to distance themselves from the mad human clamour. They communicated only with themselves, their books and God. Books gave them great consolation, and if the books were taken away, there always remained the sky, the earth and the seas; reading the book of nature attuned them to the greatness of creation.

Among the ancient exemplary figures, Cato (apparently the elder) was mentioned as a virtuous man who never listened to his slanderers, even though he was not physically deaf (p. 618). When someone apologised to him for insulting words and ridicule, Cato merely answered: "Hercules, I never noticed anything!" Cato's virtue was in not responding to scorn and resisting participation in mockery, as if he were deaf and unable to understand the slanderers. Archimedes was equally virtuous: occupied with drawing geometric circles, he failed to notice the arrival of the enemy – despite the shouts of women and dying children around him – until a soldier held a sword to his neck (p. 620). Ignorance was here a privilege given to the deaf, and even hearers should imitate such unawareness and indifference to the world. By referring to Cato and Archimedes, Schoock noted that deafness was compensated for by learning. The gift of deafness was given by God, who closed men's ears in order to protect the soul's integrity from disturbing influences and to allow peaceful conditions for concentrating on meditations of eternity.[26] As Balde concisely put it, a deaf man ignored all things (*Surdus praeterit omnia; Silvarum libri* 5.15).

Schoock further praised deaf people's ability to read human gestures and interpret emotions successfully through nearly unnoticeable physical signs. Small gestures, the movement of a finger, for example, often passed unnoticed but could be an important indicator of a secret thought (p. 621). Christian Lange, a professor of medicine at Leipzig, celebrated the thumb for similar reasons, noting how it reacted according to the human will. The thumb's upward or downward position indicated either favour or disfavour in ancient times, and it was used in threatening gestures as well (1688, Ch. XXII). In addition, Lange also praised honey used as a drug (Ch. XXIII) and the eel (Ch. XVII), called the "Helen of dinners".

As a positive example of deafness, Schoock used a tribe living near the cataracts of the Nile (p. 620). The roar of the rushing waters prevented all verbal communication in the village, but the inhabitants had learned to make themselves understood through gestures. Schoock thus slightly modified the story told by Seneca in his epistle (56.3) where Seneca too mentioned the tribe that had inhabited the cataract area, but had then moved into a city to avoid the din of rushing water. Seneca had stressed the necessity of silence for study and emphasised the importance of concentration and seclusion to maintain inner peace. In the Dream of Scipio (*De re publica* 6.18.19), Cicero had also mentioned the place called Catadupa where the Nile rushes down and the people living there had lost their sense of hearing. In the same way, Cicero argues, people have become deaf to the music of the spheres, which cannot be perceived by human ears.

But not even silence was always an unambiguously good sign. In the same epistle (56.7–8), Seneca pointed to an unfortunate fellow who had ordered total silence in his household. His servants had gone completely noiseless and walked on tip-toe. Yet the man complained about disturbing noises. In Seneca's words, the uproar of his unbalanced soul was the source of the disquiet, nothing else. When a man has learned to concentrate on good thoughts and the mind is stable, no outward noise, chance sounds, bird song, flattering words or verbal threats could interrupt or shake its peace, since all sounds were equally meaningless, like the dashing of waves or the lashing wind (Seneca, *Epistulae* 83.7). Seneca's letter 56 closed by reminding the reader of the simple cure Ulysses had found for siren song.

Seneca's *Epistles* formed a crucial subtext for these later paradoxical discussions of the good life. Already Petrarch's *De vita solitaria* (1346) was crammed with quotations from Seneca in arguing in favour of the leisurely life. Whereas the *otiosus* slept well, enjoyed silence and bird song and read for hours, the *occupatus* was always restless, deafened by chatter and urban noises and constantly troubled by anxiety. Petrarch's apology for solitude contained satirical criticism of the anxious and exhaustive urban life (Barbour 2004, p. 45; Panizza 1985, p. 197); this criticism was already familiar from Roman verse satire. Schoock's treatise too can be placed in the long tradition of satirical and philosophical works discussing the opposition between the active and the contemplative life and arguing in favour of the tranquillity of the mind.

On the wonderful lethargy

Like blindness, sleep has often been interpreted metaphorically and equated with unawareness or forgetfulness. Just as there were degrees in the injuriousness of the diseases according to the body parts they affected, disorders of the head – the instrument of judgement and cognitive faculty – were considered worse, owing to their site on the body. These disorders included lethargies, migraines, epilepsies, apoplexies and fevers that escalated the pitch of delirium.[27] They rendered the patient unable to perceive his sick condition, and in the eyes of the satirists this unawareness was usually more fatal than other diseases. In his *Miscellanea curiosa medica*, Christian Lange cited Seneca's epistle (53.7), which noted that the worse the disease of the soul, the less we notice it (1688, Ch. X). Seneca compared this lack of self-knowledge to sleep and slumber, which sink the spirit so deep that it has no perception of self. A sleeping person was associated with a sinner who failed to recognise the faults of his spirit. Aware and awake were two names given to the same phenomenon, self-recognition. Seneca had underlined the duty and force of philosophy as "the only power that can shake off our deep slumber" (53.8; trans. Richard M. Gummere). Seneca also wrote that even sick men should be congratulated if they perceived their own sickness (6.1).

In Roman satire sleepiness also provided an analogy for unawareness of the self. One of the key symptoms of the ailing mind in Persius' third satire was the patient's physical and moral somnolence. Reckford, describing Persius' lethargic patient, writes that he is "so relaxed, in fact, that his head almost falls off; he snores so violently that his jaws become loosened" (1998, pp. 344–5).[28] The point of this description was the author's wake-up call to study philosophy instead of wasting his life. In his commentary on Persius' third satire, Johannes Murmellius saw that the satirist's target was the inactivity and idleness of rich, noble young men, since for the students of the trivium arts, three things were necessary: vigilance, avoidance of excessive attention to the body, and simple nourishment (1516, xxi^{v}). Likewise, in Horace's satire (2.3) arousing the drowsy mind from its deep lethargy (*lethargus grandis*) was the satirist's duty. The doctor in this passage was pessimistic about the human mind; as a quick thinker and a loyal friend, as Horace put it, the doctor ordered a table to be brought in and poured out there some bags of coins to awaken the patient from a coma (2.3.145–57). In Landino's view (1486, *ad loc.*), the reason for the doctor's action was his awareness of the man's fundamental avarice. Landino noted in this passage that lethargy meant oblivion, as though a frenetic patient was unwilling to see a doctor. Horace himself reported having great difficulties falling asleep, even though he had an oil massage, soaked himself in strong wine and counted the triumphs of Caesar (*Sermones* 2.1.7–11). This wakefulness ironically bespoke the satirist's heightened awareness, in contrast to his drowsy patients.[29]

As a general metaphor for the vices of sloth, sluggishness and laziness, sleepiness was deeply opposite the philosophical and satirical ideals of self-awareness and keen perception of truth. Satires were often written precisely against men's lethargy and as wake-up-calls to virtue and energetic labour. In Boethius's *De consolatione philosophiae*, the personified Philosophy told the narrator that his illness was caused by his lethargy, which was a common disease (I.2.5, *lethargum patitur, communem illusarum mentium morbum*), and forgetfulness, that he did not remember who he really was (I.6.17). There was no cure for a disease that was not understood, and lack of self-knowledge was the greatest cause of the narrator's disease. Philosophy presented herself as a doctor, who made the diagnosis of lethargy or stupor, and the remedy was found in reason and self-knowledge. Joel C. Relihan considered this view of wisdom characteristic of consolatory discourse in general (2007, pp. 5, 53). In this tradition, poet and theologian Johann Sebastian Wieland (1590–1635), for example, called his satirical poem *melissa*, this being in his words a miraculous medicinal plant that sharpened the mind, purged the ears and brightened the eyes by healing the glaucoma of envy (1618b). The purpose of his healing poem was to expel lethargy (*lethargum expellens*) and provoke the reader to undertake hard work and vigilance through satirical virtue.

Another negative image linked sleep with death (Vredeveld 2001, p. 874; Franck 1681, §43–9). The famous epic story of the siren song concretely combined these two phenomena, when music's dangerous power made the sailors drowsy and caused their ships to be dashed upon the rocks. Homer also spoke of sleep as death's brother, their shared ancestry being recognised in that there was no sensation in either and both brought calm rest (*Iliad* 14.231; cf. Cicero, *Tusc.* 1.38.92). But sleep and death were also paradoxically praised in that they liberated men from the world of distress and all the evils of mankind. Rhetorician Alcidamas was famous for writing an encomium of death in which he listed the evils to which the living were exposed (Cicero, *Tusc.* 1.48.116). Sleep came as a relief to men who were consumed by worries and worldly cares. Satirists such as Codrus Urceus declared that even death did not bring solace to men who had sinned, since they have to pay for their deeds in the Underworld (1506, *sat.* 1–2).

It is known in the history of mock-encomia that it was probably Fronto who wrote a praise to insomnia, but usually the genre turned the conventional negative association of sleepiness around and eulogised it. This approach was supported by empirical facts and medical views, which reported on the restorative physical benefits of sleep. A proper amount of sleep was a traditional issue in medical literature, and doctors saw that good sleep and health were related. Georg Franck von Franckenau noted in his dissertation *Quam diu dormiendum* (1681) that moderate sleep was praised with good reason by ancient poets and later physicians as well, since it refreshed the mind, rendered active capacities livelier, sharpened the sense perceptions, increased the temperature of the intestines and thereby advanced digestion and urged the blood to circulate rapidly. It also soothed pain, calmed the mind and abolished distress and worries.[30] Similar views were expressed by Daniel Sennert (1628, p. 863, *De somno et vigiliis*) and according to Christian Lange (1688, Ch. X), sleep was especially important for gout patients, who were often afflicted by constant pains and insomnia. Sweet sleep tamed the lion, that is, alleviated even severe pain. It reintegrated physical strength, improved the health and dispelled excess fluids from the body. Sleep was here paradoxically discussed in terms that indicated its rational and harmonising impact on humans: sleep was a doctor that restored men to work. In Lange's words, Orpheus rightly saluted Somnus as the king of the blessed gods and all mortal beings. Franck noted that Synesius in *De insomniis* and Tertullian in his *Liber de anima* (cap. 43, *De somno*) had called sleep a doctor (*medicus laborum*) as well. Through references to ancient poetry Franck inferred that sleep was omnipotent.[31]

Franck also appreciated the dangers of insomnia – used as a means of torture in Java, for example – and knew of curious cases where people had stayed awake for months after having overindulged in drinking tea or, in the case of manic patients, even for years, the record being 35 years of wakefulness experienced by a noble lady. The other extreme was lethargy and excessive sleepiness, likened to death by many ancient authors, and the analogy was discussed here as well. Franck recorded tales told of long-sleeping historical and mythical figures. For example, a group of inebriated young men had slept in Athens for four days; a German peasant slept over the winter in a haystack; a schoolboy from Lübeck was asleep for seven years and did not age, and a shepherd, Epimenides Gnosius, slept for 75 years in a cave in Crete. In one of the most unusual cases ever to occur, seven young men of Ephesus, fleeing the persecutions of the Christians, escaped to the mountains where they slept for 196 years.[32] Another seven men slept on an Atlantic island for centuries and if someone touched them his limbs dried up. The reasons given for the extraordinary length of sleep varied from natural causes to demons and the punishment of God. Usually, in medical literature both insomnia and lethargy were considered pathological states. Daniel Sennert defined lethargy a chronic urge to sleep, accompanied by oblivion of all things and mild fever (1628, pp. 312–14, 330, 399 and 458).

Considering the amount of attention given to the issue in medical literature, it is no surprise to find that sleep was also treated in panegyrics. Christoph Hegendorff's (1500–40) *Encomium somni* (1519) was a ironic monologue given by the figure Somnus.[33] Following the conventions of epideictic rhetoric, the speech began by examining his ancestry: his father was Night; his mother Lethe; and his sisters, Analysis, Phantasia and Onar. The six-page-long speech concentrated on the power of Sleep to appease anger, restlessness and worries. These all were emotions that made life unhappy in some way. Recurrent waves of anger prohibited rational thinking, and sleep was often the only means to calm the mind. If in the evening the mind was perturbed by the strong emotions of anger and envy, in the morning it felt only regret, owing to a night of good sleep. Thus, sleep helped to maintain friendly relations between men and restored positive feelings.

The speech further described how people seemed who were oppressed by worries or too much philosophical reading: having lost their sense of humour, their faces turned sour, wrinkles on their foreheads deepened and the crowns of their heads grew bald. Salutary sleep cured all unhealthy symptoms and recalled a youthful spirit, so that after a night of good sleep, the body returned to its earlier resplendence. Many of the benefits produced by sleep seemed to parallel philosophical and Stoic goals: a reduction of passions, the faculty of rational thinking and tranquillity of mind. Moreover, sleep relieved hangovers and restored the drinker's ability to work. It also shared many features with personified diseases, for example, the omnipotence familiar from gout eulogies. Sleep was here called both a doctor and a remedy, and it adopted the medico-philosophical tasks of consolation and bringing healthy balance to the disturbed mind.

Hegendorff's encomium also made sleep a consolation for poor people. Plutarch, for example, had noted that the balm of sleep made slaves forget their masters, reduced the weight of prisoners' chains and soothed the pain caused by inflammation and gnawing ulcers ("Superstition", *Moralia* 165E). It was a gift of forgetfulness bestowed by the gods. Likewise, Hegendorff stressed that those who had hard times in real life could, while asleep, dream of wealth and gold and imagine themselves to be the famous rich men, Croesus and Crassus. Even those who considered committing suicide were often dissuaded from such calamitous plans when night turned to morning. While asleep, they were freed from all agitation. Other benefits of sleep included the nightly omens revealed to the sleeping, the prevention of serious diseases and the consolation and refreshment given to travellers. The short speech closed with a poem in which Endymion, addressing his words to Sleep, repeated some of the benefits already mentioned.

As Annette Tomarken has noted (1990, p. 255, n. 17), even though Hegendorff's eulogy was often found bound into medical tracts, it was a typical mock encomium. Shorter poems on night and sleep were also included in Dornau's compilation (1619, pp. 718–19). Hegendorff's eulogy also had certain affinities with the elegiac and religious poetry that lamented the burden of earthly living and the distress and restlessness caused by human worries or by metaphysical anxieties. In such poems, usually addressed to Sleep, the poet invoked and prayed to sleep as a spirit of eternity to free him of his burden and to sooth him with its gentle spirit into pleasurable unawareness and insensibility. Sleep was a condition in which the poet gained a welcome distance from the human world and forgot his pains and worries, which were often described as "sleepless". Or sleep was the spirit of the divine healer whom the Christian poet awaited to redeem him. In these poems, insomnia and sound sleep represented two kinds of life, suffering and happiness (Häussler 1978, p. 121).

Among the early modern Neo-Latin sleep elegies, mention can be made of the elegy *Ad somnum* by Sidronius De Hossche (1596–1653), often regarded as one of the greatest Jesuit Latin poets. It began with a conventional invocation to the god of sleep, asking him to come "and with gentle wings fan lightly / My tired eyes which long for sleep" (trans. James J. Mertz *et al.*). Sleep was invited to restore new strength to the poet, stop all tears, ease the heart of grief and scatter worries. Yet at the end of the elegy the sleep turned into a cruel and iron-cold spirit, the image of death, which the poet commanded to stay far from him. Instead, the poet chose life.[34] Jacob Balde also dedicated an ode to sleep, *Ad somnum*, calling sleep "death's gentle brother", asking sleep to come and flow through his limbs like healing oil and bring morning freshness and new strength. Sleep was here opposed to the heavy tedium that had taken a firm hold of the poet. Balde's satirical and playful spirit was shown in his repeated requests that sleep would enter without heavy snoring, a symptom that had, in Persius' third satire, meant profound unconsciousness. Here the coarse sound of the mere word *rhonchus* provided comic relief, which broke the serious spirit of lamentation and restored the poet to life and laughter.[35]

The ambivalence of intoxication

Although not actually a sensory disability, the state of drunkenness was capable of producing wonderful unawareness and deep sleep as well. Because several paradoxical eulogies were devoted to this issue, one which affected all the senses as well as the cognitive faculty, I will conclude this chapter with a brief treatment of drunkenness. Tomarken, among others, has noted, "no sin has so rich a literature in the sixteenth century as drunkenness" (1990, p. 52). Satirists and other moralists produced numerous works levelling charges against inebriation as a state that reduced men to beasts. They filled their verses and pages intended to criticise gluttony with colourful descriptions of drinking bouts and drunken bodies. For example, Balde laconically inquired how anyone's aim in life could be drinking, vomiting and filling himself with food (1651, *sat.* 3). The subtitle of Johann Sebastian Wieland's *Amethystus* (1618) identified the poem as a sober satire directed against a drunken cohort and indeed, the poem consisted of attacks on gluttony and drinking. The poem strongly echoed Roman verse satire, and in the manner of Juvenal's first poem protested the poet's silence, claiming that it was difficult to remain a passive listener when such a number of vices and the dirt of luxury was around every day (A3). Anger gnawed at the poet's dry liver (A4), as it had done in Juvenal's poem (1.45). Wieland recorded the horrifying effects of drinking, the irrational howling of the inebriated, the licking of the last drop (a frequent scornful image in this connection), the consequent social ills like quarrels and the unnatural changes in character caused by drinking, so that a man normally more silent than a pupil from Samos turned to rioting, making more noise than the breaking waves or the birds from Daulia, the scene of the tragic story of Philomela and Procne (A3). The poem contained a number of images familiar from Roman satire, from sour belches arising from the belly to the superb men dressed in hyacinthine cloaks and conspicuous jewel rings; it included their heavy snoring when they fell asleep only to wake up again and continue their former conduct. These images were familiar from Persius' poetry. There was nothing ambivalent or approving in these attacks; drunken men were explicitly called Epicurean swine and condemned. The poem deserves attention here, because it also contained a long passage describing various diseases resulting from illicit living (A7v): "Most of the sick drinkers die, since the undigested food stagnates in the ardent stomach and creates languor. This gives rise to a wealth of diseases." The pathological features diagnosed resembled the self-induced diseases and the disabilities familiar from Roman satire and other morally critical contexts: dimmed and aching eyes that were anointed in vain, if the patient did not amend the whole course of his life; half-deaf ears; gout; scabies and *morbus regius*; phthisis and vomiting.

Similar lists recording diseases that originated in inebriation were frequently encountered in these connections. Vincentius Obsopoeus's (d. 1539) art of drinking, *De arte bibendi*, mentioned chronic pains, lost vigour in the limbs, vertigo, permanent facial pallor, trembling hands, fingers contorted by chiragra, dim and reddish eyes, stomach ache, tinnitus, battalions of fevers, scabies, dropsy, breaths as foul as those arising from public sewers, mental rabies and fury, and, finally, premature old age and sudden deaths intestate (pp. 39–40). These were not only actual symptoms of heavy and continual drinking, but also emphatically moral and pathological signs reminding one of the diagnoses made in Roman satire, for example, in Juvenal's tenth satire, which described the illnesses that took place in old age. The moralising descriptions thus had a recognisable literary background that was repeatedly recalled in the tradition of satire. In *Jus potandi*, hangover and vomiting were also described as diseased conditions (I.60).

Vivid characterisations of drunken bodies were a way of showing one's rhetorical vigour and were part of the satirist's arsenal of playful attacks. One professor of rhetoric, Georgius Nicolasius (1590–1621), delivered a speech in 1620 entitled *Methigraphia*, which concentrated on the effects of drinking. In the beginning he excused his aggressive tone in an already familiar apology (albeit with a somewhat clumsy allusion to hurting), explaining that he had thrown a stone for the sake of sanity, to make a patient recognise his illness and heal him (p. 2). The patient was a man who, in his insatiability, was well on the way to metamorphosing into an amphora. Different metamorphoses – usually from men to animals – caused by drinking were recorded in a number of similar texts. Here the roundness of the vessel nicely captured the drinker's chubby appearance. His cheeks swelled and the parturient stomach began to rumble and utter sounds suggesting an approaching storm (p. 4).

The belly's swellings and a-foot-and-a-half-long expressions (*sesquipedalia verba*) consisted of genuine liquid and slimy sounds finally picked up, as a concrete substance, by swine and dogs. Nicolasius's description of the complaining stomach was rhetorically composed of multiple and not always smoothly running figurative layers and quasi-Horatian expressions that referred to the creation of a disappointing result, an over-elaborate speech produced by the belly that the animals then devoured. Special attention was given to the sounds and fragrances elicited by the bowels. They were compared with different harsh sounds that had an unpleasant acoustic effect: explosives, catapults and other flying and aerial weapons (p. 13). When drunk people also elicited raucous animal voices, scholastic syllogisms and dissertations, and words of abuse, blasphemy and other forms of verbal roughness (p. 14). Finally, when released from the bodily cavities the hot vapour acquired the forces of mere fury, insanity and alienation of the mind (p. 13).

Other effects ensuing from the drinking included various diseases, the indigestion of an ever-full stomach and over-nutrition. Nicolasius mentioned premature senility, vertigo, stupor and dullness of the head, dimness of the eyes caused by the crude fluids that tried to find an exit, foul-smelling breath arising from the suffering inside, the cruel goddess gout, dropsy and other internal plagues (p. 9). The moral failures had their seats within the man, as they had had in Roman satire, but Nicolasius elaborated especially on the scatological possibilities of the imagery.

The Greeks had personified the god of wine in the figure of Bacchus, but the early modern moralising poems imagined instead a goddess of inebriation, Ebrietas or (more intimately) Ebria. The satirist Nicodemus Frischlin composed a well-known and often reprinted elegy against inebriation, in which he introduced Ebrietas as a triumphal goddess living in the northern region near the Rhine (1615, pp. 66–7). Like the goddess Podagra, Ebrietas was also accompanied by different personified vices like physical love, blasphemy, outspokenness, anger, lust, fury and deceit. Her appearance suggested the effects of inveterate alcoholism, with her greenish skin colour, putrid ulcers, cheeks hanging loose like a mantle, foul breath that was like bad air arising from the earth, rotten teeth and trembling hands. Moreover, she was completely naked and dishonourable.

Obsopoeus's *De arte bibendi* and its description of the garden of Ebria offered a very similar allegorical vision (1648, pp. 25–7). The goddess's suite included the personified Dementia, Luxury, Oblivion, Idleness, Languor, Quarrels, Insanity, Rabies and Fury. This party was accompanied by different beasts, bears, asses, sheep, goats, wolves, bulls and swine – all former men metamorphosed into animals by reason of their drinking. They suffered from the same diseases that were repeatedly found and related above in the description of drunken people, including lethargy, wounds, pallor and fever (p. 27). They even absorbed their own vomiting like dogs (p. 35).[36]

But sometimes the conventional vices of drunkenness and gluttony, instead of being attacked as vices and human errors, were welcomed as conducive to the overall sanity of the body and the mind. Paradox, one of the favourite devices of perception and argumentation in the seventeenth century, was again used here, when the favourable effects of drinking wine were highlighted. Wine was one of the most ancient remedies for strengthening body and soul and for regulating the temperamental quality of the humours, something the satirists never forgot. An anecdote in *Nugae venales* recommended drinking wine on the basis that "Hippocrates and Galen had called it a first-rate medicament that gave comfort, warmed the frigid nerves, purged melancholy, provoked urine, warmed the stomach, suppressed vomiting and encouraged men to heroic deeds" (pp. 6–7). Obsopoeus urged men to drink at home, where peace and love reigned, and drinking acquired the status of a private pleasure; outside the home it often brought disagreement and quarrels (1648, pp. 2–5). Obsopoeus composed a eulogy to Bacchus and thanked him for investing men with the virtue of courage, giving them hope, restoring vigour in their limbs, comforting them in their sadness, calming them down, wiping away their tears, making poor conditions seem bearable and bringing sweet dreams and oblivion to everything (p. 21). Intoxication here had consolatory and recreational effects very similar to beneficial sleep.[37]

In other humorous and satirical discussions about the favourable and less beneficial effects of drinking wine, very similar arguments were used. Filippo Beroaldo dealt with the benefits and disadvantages of drinking in a dialogue among three brothers – a fornicator, a gambler and a drunkard (*Quaestio quis inter scortatorem, aleatorem & ebriosum sit pessimus*, 1499). The dialogue was constructed like a trial scene, in which the brothers defended themselves in order to show who was the least immoral and thus the legitimate heir to their father's entire legacy. Authorities like Plato, Seneca and Asclepiades were recalled by the drunken son as having recommended the use of wine, for it made the mind sharper and the tongue smoother. Heracles, Alexander the Great and even the severe and wise Cato were known to have used wine (p. 141). The mention of Cato is meant to appear surprising and paradoxical, since he was represented by Horace (*Epistulae* 1.19.12–14) as abstemious and not an authority to suggest that men should drink deeply. The greatest benefit offered by wine was that it wiped away the feelings of sadness, anxiety and other diseases from the mind. It brought sweet oblivion, happiness (*vita beata*), security and tranquillity – ideals that the Stoics greatly appreciated. In the drinker's words, Bacchus was not called Liber because of his loose tongue and frankness, but because he freed the mind from its bondage to cares (p. 140).

In Beroaldo's dialogue the other two sons strongly doubted the ability of wine to produce positive mental effects. By appealing to physical and mental health as the most precious things in human life, they reminded their brother that health was in fact often violated by drinking (p. 144). The mind was clouded and physical strength diminished, and these were followed by loss of reputation. An etymological counterargument was used: wine was called *temetum*, since it had a firm hold on the mind (*teneat mentem*). Thus, drinking brought with it the vice of self-ignorance that was so strongly condemned by the philosophers; it also had other detrimental effects specifically on the mind. Instead of the ideal situation, whereby reason commanded the body, fatuity, oblivion and other mental failures ensued when wine led the mind, as if in a voluntary insanity (pp. 145–6). Sweet oblivion of all things was here considered negative; a man did not even remember death – which, of course, was a major failure, considering that philosophers often saw the whole purpose of philosophy as the preparation of man for death. Familiar, morally associated diseases (ulcers, resolution of the nerves, trembling hands, fevers and gout) were mentioned. The ill effects also included the resulting social vices: fights, murders and thefts (p. 148). As an argument against drinking, ancient examples were given (pp. 151–6), such as Emperor Tiberius Claudius Nero (proverbially known as "Biberius Claudius Mero"); the Spartans who made their slaves drink wine, then sent them to young people's drinking parties as warning examples of shameful behaviour; and ancient Egyptian priests and Carthaginian soldiers who drank only water to keep their senses clear.

Intoxication thus caused several passions and vices, including anger and lust, that philosophy struggled to prevent and control. It caused shameful changes in people's character; Lot even had sexual affairs with his daughters when drunk (p. 159). This version slightly modifies the story found in Genesis 19, where Lot offered his daughters to strangers. Several ancient authorities were quoted to condemn drunkenness. According to Aesop or Anacharsis, the five toasts were the following: first to thirst, second to joy, third to pleasure, fourth to shame and finally, the fifth, to fury and insanity (p. 160). The adulterous and the gambling son also quoted a list of the physical effects of drinking, attributed to Pliny, which included once again the pallor, flagging cheeks, ulcerated eyes, trembling hands, furious dreams, foul breath, death of memory, and so on (p. 163). The arguments against inebriation were allotted a much larger space in the dialogue than those in its favour.

Drunkenness was usually recommended for the reason that it brought joy and happiness to drinkers, purified the body, removed cares, rendered the shy bold and the silent talkative. Not only were Dionysus, Bacchus and the sophisticated pleasures of drinking applauded, but so was downright intoxication. Praises of drunkenness were popular in the Renaissance, and texts entitled *artes bibendi* were written in playful imitation of didactic poetry. An example of a positive evaluation was the theoretico-practical disputation *Jus potandi* by two pseudonymous authors, the respondent Blasius Multibibus and his supervisor Dionysius Bacchus, both from the College of Hilarity. The authors went systematically through different draughts: total drinking (*totalis*), continual sips (*continuus*), drinking without breathing (*hausticus*) and a single gulp (*floricus*), which created bubbles arising in the nostrils (I.9). They also examined the positive effects of drinking, such as beautiful poetry and artful verses (*Ich fuhr mich ubern Rhein, Bonum vinum post Martinum*) and intelligent discussions about elevating topics in Latin (*De ente et essentia; Mysteria Platonica*) (I.39–41).

These arts, defences and apologies were parodical and paradoxical when compared with general moral views as well as with Stoic ethics. Chrysippus, for example, had maintained that illness could undermine the faculty of reason without the wise man consciously consenting, but drunkenness was always a man's deliberate choice and voluntary and hence, an immoral act that destroyed virtue (Ronnick 1991, p. 31). Virtue and the sense of shame were easily lost when one was inebriated, and inebriation had been a stock topic in ancient philosophical discussions about the relationship between mind and body (Tieleman 2003, pp. 163–6). Seneca discussed drunkenness in his epistle (83) and noted that Zeno discouraged men from drunkenness. By quoting Posidonius, he distinguished between two kinds of drunkenness: a man soaked in wine and having no control of himself, and a man who was a slave to his drinking habit; of these, the inveterate habit was, of course, worse. Drinking exposed a man to shameful deeds, rendered him powerless over his soul and disclosed all his vices. Although Seneca recorded here the calamities caused by drunkenness, he also remarked that wine did not necessarily create vices but rather brought them into public view.

Christoph Hegendorff was famous for his eulogy of drunkenness, which demonstrated with examples that drinking was a minor sin and had many advantages both for physical health and mental well-being. Later on, he took back his words and articulated his moral views more clearly by writing another praise, this time in defence of clear-headedness and sobriety, *Encomium sobrietatis*, in which he stressed that inebriation caused much damage and led to lies, fights and murders (Tomarken 1990, pp. 53–4).[38] In *Declamatio in laudem ebrietatis* (1526), attributed to Hegendorff and dedicated to jurist Franciscus Parcenius Soldanus as a New Year's present, the author stated that his purpose, ironically, was to praise drunkenness as a means of exercising his style and indirectly to recommend sobriety. The grounds on which he favoured drinking were based on famous ancient and biblical examples. Noah, who had his own vineyard and became intoxicated; Lot, who occasionally drank so much that he slept with his daughters (an event mentioned as though approvingly, but the remark is ironic); and Joseph and his brothers, all of whom consumed wine (aaiiij–aaiiij^{v}). Philosophical authorities and symposium literature (Plato, Plutarch) were also quoted to defend the consumption of wine, since it made these ancient men discuss serious issues. Several Roman emperors were known for this habit, and even Cato, the most notable censor of manners, excelled in this art. Inebriation was adored as a god among the Spanish and Egyptian peoples, and all other countries shared this predilection, which was in fact universal (aa5^{v}–aa6).

Nature was referred to here as a model that directed men to use wine. Significantly, Hegendorff applied medical arguments as well: it was noted that drinking was a salutary thing, good for physical health and for easing pain (aa7). Drinking also served the traditional role of philosophy in curing pestilential diseases of the mind: the drinker forgot his troubles, and even if they were not completely extirpated, at least they were made tolerable and softened. The etymology of Bacchus' name was also mentioned here; he liberated the mind from worries, sorrows and mental disorders (aa7^{v}). Sober people were troubled by insomnia, and constant reminders of their grief kept them awake around the clock. Wine, by contrast, made even the poor happy, since their hardships, debts and difficulties in making a living did not weigh on their minds when they slept (aa8). Even the monks could stand their poor living conditions by force of these noble drinks. Thus, delight and happiness were among the positive consequences of drinking, as seen on in the beer labelled Gaudium (aa8). Ironically, Hegendorff noted that when the blind, the mute or the lame were gathered together on St Peter's and St Paul's marketplace near Leipzig, their condition was conspicuously improved when they were given food and drink. The blind man no longer needed a guide, the lame danced and the mute communicated through gestures (aa8^{v}). Even if their disabilities did not completely disappear, they were made endurable, which proved the healthiness of drinking.

According to Hegendorff, other benefits included an improved faculty of eloquence, so that even silent peasants demonstrated through their lively talk that they differed from the animals. The effect of increased fluency was noted in bridal parties, and poets and apostles were inspired by wine, without which they were unable to create anything elegant, beautiful or durable (bb–bb^{v}). In addition to gracefulness, wine produced truthfulness as well: there was no need to torture criminals to get information, when the simple offer of wine was enough to loosen their tongues. People's secret thoughts and private manners were revealed by this simple trick (bbij). Hegendorff's declamation closed with authoritative quotations from the Bible, meant to persuade the audience that neither Jesus, Moses nor St Paul in fact condemned the drinking of wine, since wine was a gift of God; they only objected to harmful excessive inebriation, which was not beneficial to the human mind (bbij^{v}–bbiiij).

These satirical discussions of the effects of drunkenness on men's health were ambivalent. A vast number of satires recorded the full horror of the diseased condition that resulted from shameful drinking, the most prominent vice attacked in the early modern texts. On the other hand, this moral criticism was at times turned around, when the benefits of drinking were assessed by appealing to improved physical health, the recreation of the mind, and the wonderful obliviousness to all troubles and cares. Intoxication served as a consolation against any hardship, re-educated the patient as did philosophy and restored the drunkard's intellectual abilities. The words used here for the results of drinking were familiar from the philosophical discussions of the good life, including happiness and tranquillity of mind. Parodically exaggerating philosophical and consolatory discourse, the author of *Declamatio in laudem ebrietatis* presented drinking in a positive light without abandoning the satirical aim of playful moral discussion.

But while praising the indefensible object, the writers always kept a sense of irony, mockery and ridicule in the air. Therefore, it is at times difficult to decide if their paradoxical praise was meant to argue seriously that the object praised was better than usually thought or if, beneath its eloquent guise, was merely confirming conventional values and the vileness of the object. Although the disease eulogies were usually written from a Stoic perspective, with pain despised and men advised to devote their sick leave to studying Stoic wisdom, one can also doubt the sincerity of their instruction. What if the authors were in fact ironic Epicureans? We know that Balde, who also wrote a satire about the misuse of tobacco (*Satyra contra abusum tabaci*, 1657), was himself an addicted smoker (Knepper 1904, p. 59). One can also ask whether it was at all possible to defend and praise something that was conventionally considered to be of little value or even harmful. When praising dwarfs in his speech of 1599, did Albert Wichgreve manage to save them from contempt and scorn? Or was it just a clever disguise for conventional aesthetics, in which deformity – either physical ugliness or mental ignorance – was still the primary source of ridicule? Nevertheless, satirical eulogies testify to the ability of language to magnify a thing by praising it or diminish it by censuring. In their capacity to change perspectives, both satire (making great things small) and paradox (making small things great) can be read as expressions that question the conventional value of health, beauty and wealth and show us that excessive wealth and constant health can also induce sloth and other vices.

5
Outlook and Virtue: Morally Symptomatic Physical Peculiarities

In the previous chapters, it has been repeatedly noted that satirical authors and philosophers alike have elaborated on the idea that physical appearance and the condition of the body have moral significance. The human face, for example, was thought to express a person's deeper moral qualities. Cicero viewed impudence as a disease discernable on a man's face and in his gait, and Jerome called the face, whose silent eyes were capable of disclosing the secrets of the heart, the mirror of the mind (Mancinellus and Badius Ascensius 1515, fol. xx^{r}). In his *Apocolocyntosis* Seneca also famously depicted the Emperor Claudius as a vile body, whose infirmities directly reflected his moral dissolution (cf. Braund and James 1998); meanwhile, the appearance and gait of Maecenas revealed his degeneration (*Epistulae* 114.4). In the Juvenalian saying, anguish and pleasure stamp themselves on the visage (2.17, *vultu morbum incessuque fatetur*; cf. 9.18–20). Early modern satirists printed out the same revealing signs. Petrus Cunaeus's Menippean satire *Sardi venales* deplored the universal sickness of his time when "everybody confessed their illnesses by their countenance and gait" (1620, p. 65).

On the other hand, satires often also constructed an opposition between the false first appearance and the true inner side of human beings. In his satire *Arx virtutis,* Havraeus expressed this conventional contrast, saying that a slow gait and a timid outlook did not necessarily reflect a man's character; on the contrary, such things could well conceal a generous mind and the courage of a lion (1627, *sat.* 2). Havraeus borrowed these expressions from Roman verse satire – another Juvenalian saying was "never trust the front" – and he elaborated on ancient phrases taken from Juvenal, Virgil and Cicero that had warned of secret evils: roses had thorns, serpents hid in the grass, the firm gait could deceive; for many men simulation and pretence were the whole of life.

Whatever conclusion was reached about a man's moral condition on the basis of his appearance, it always remained morally relevant and the locus of the satirists' keen interest. Therefore, it is tempting to ask could any physical sign whatsoever acquire morally significant meanings? I would answer in the affirmative; there seemed to be no physical feature or symptom that could not be morally interpreted in satires. In addition to realistically depicted sick, drunken and vice-laden bodies, which openly revealed a man's immorality, early modern satires also recognised a number of more imaginative case records and surprising symptoms. The following discussion will focus on eulogies that can loosely be classified as belonging to the subgenre of satirical encomia that deal with physical peculiarities, deformities and curiosities. According to Tomarken, physical strangeness was satirically praised, especially in sixteenth-century France (1990, p. 167), but similar Neo-Latin works were produced in other countries as well. They eulogised physical peculiarities and qualities that were not usually regarded as beautiful or desirable and that differed from the common standards of bodily perfection. Humorous body parts – the nose and the lower parts – had a firm place in this genre. Evaluation of mental and sexual vigour from the size of the nose was, of course, commonplace; its magnitude could, for example, reveal man's capacity for acting like an emperor (*Nugae venales*, p. 18). Another anecdote contained the following praise of the rear end:

> Master *hinterland* excels all other body parts in dignity. First of all, he is a veritable *philosopher*, because he has a beard. Secondly, he is a significant *advocate*, which is proved by the clarity and frankness with which he pronounces his inner thoughts to such an extent that no other advocate dares to move his nose. Thirdly, he is a fearless *captain*, who clearly either wants to conquer or to be conquered or killed, he fights so furiously. Fourthly, he is an extremely charitable *peasant*, who often manures his neighbour's fields for nothing. Fifthly, he is an excellent *artist*, who rapidly adumbrates various figures in the clothes or in the linen as soon as the bed is made. [...] Seventh, he is a first-class *musician*. Even though divine and vocal music is charming, it cannot compete with the music of the arse, since vocal music merely touches the sense of hearing, but this music delights all five senses of hearing, smell, taste, sight and touch [...]. (*Nugae venales*, pp. 16–17, *Recita laudes podicis*)

Similar organic music, distinguished from harmonic music, was praised in the pseudo-scientific discussion of farting, *De peditu*. In this category of paradoxical praises can also be included praise of baldness (in imitation of Synesius' *Calvitii encomium*), the beard,[1] horns,[2] ugly faces, fatness or thinness and many physical eccentricities such as praise of dwarfs. The triviality of the subject under consideration was denied on the basis that it could be connected to several remarkable men from the past. Synesius defended baldness by asserting that the noblest ancient men – priests and philosophers – were hairless. In *Barbae maiestas* (1614) the same argument was used about the beard: it was a natural ornament and a distinguishing mark that decorated the cheeks of Jesus and St. Peter, as leaves adorn trees; wool, the lambs; and feathers, the birds (p. 6). Wearing a beard was also healthful, because by absorbing excess fluids, it kept the teeth in good condition and protected the face both from burning sun and biting cold (p. 10). However, in his consolatory poem *Carmen Saturnalitium*, Balde consoled a beardless friend and reminded him that wearing a beard made men look like lustful goats, highwaymen or the fauns (*Lyricorum libri* 1.20).

Encomiasts sought for arguments that proved the usefulness and value of seemingly useless and vile things, and selected and expanded upon favourable facts while neglecting less complimentary information (Tomarken 1990, pp. 55–6). In his *Ars rhetorica*, Aristides noted four characteristic methods of praise: exaggeration of meritorious details, suppression of the undesirable, favourable contrasts and the clever turning of the unpleasant into something pleasant (Pease 1926, p. 37). The texts analysed below offer examples of all these devices. In addition to eulogies, several quasi-scientific dissertations were also devoted to strange diseases and their moral relevance.

Albert Wichgreve's praise of dwarfs

Albert Wichgreve's (1575–1619) little-known speech entitled *Oratio pro Μικανθρωποις sive homullis* (Oration in Favour of Small People) was delivered in Rostock around 1599 at a university festival organised by the Rector of Rostock University, Wilhelm Lauremberg. Wichgreve was a poet and teacher in Hamburg who studied theology and philology, earned a degree in philosophy at Wittenberg, taught at Rostock from 1597 as a *Privatdozent* and from 1605 served as a preacher in Allermöhe near Hamburg. His most famous literary work was a Latin comedy on student life, *Cornelius relegatus*. In his speech on small people, Wichgreve praised dwarfs and presented the great advantages and all possible positive sides – both moral and practical – of shortness, brevity and being small. The speech was included in the *Facetiae facetiarum* of 1627, where the full title declared that the texts included were pleasurable and useful moral reading. Wichgreve himself numbered his speech among such satirical works as Johann Fischart's *Aller Practiken Grossmutter, Asinus avis, De hasione, De crepitu ventris* and Dedekind's *Grobianus,* and he referred to Lucian, Synesius, Erasmus and Favorinus as his predecessors (pp. 13–14). Wichgreve's speech is analysed here in more detail because of its playfully ethical content and the strong emphasis it placed on the virtues of the mind in contrast to the body – features that all the satirical texts studied here have shared.

Wichgreve's topic was even more paradoxical in his day than it may seem now, because since antiquity, physical deformity has been regarded as being among the principal targets of scorn. In classical rhetoric, ugliness and physical deformity frequently produced material for jokes (Cicero, *De oratore* 2.239), and laughter was usually understood as scornful and contemptuous, laughing at someone. Deformed slaves and misshapen dwarfs were very popular in antiquity and were on display at the Emperor's court (Garland 1995, pp. 46–8). As Barry Sanders has observed (1995, pp. 209–19), during the Renaissance jokebooks poked fun at the disabled. Kings still kept dwarfs for purposes of entertainment, and their humiliation provided amusement at dinner parties and other festive occasions. This fascination has been explained later through a superiority theory: the owner of a misshapen dwarf felt satisfaction in being elevated and placed above his pet. Thomas Hobbes memorably argued in his *Leviathan* that people were fascinated with the handicapped and the deformed, because they reminded men of their own well-being. Hobbes defined this feeling as a sudden glory, which captivated any one of us on seeing misshapen individuals. In the later sixteenth century, standards of good taste gradually affected humour, and it became socially unacceptable to laugh at deformities. According to Sanders, taste, decorum and politeness forbade aristocrats to ridicule dwarfs, but this type of humour still survived in jokebooks and collections of anecdotes, which were widely read in private.

Wichgreve took a different attitude to deformity and dwarfs in his speech; instead of poking fun, he singled out the great advantages of being small and dwarfed. These qualities were fine objects for paradoxical praise, since the purpose of epideictic rhetoric was to make the object seem great, laudable and desirable, for which the dwarfs offered, of course, a suitable challenge. In panegyrics the virtuous quality of the person praised was reflected in his physical appearance: in his upright character, noble gait, strong limbs and dignified countenance, all of which expressed his moral vigour and humanity. Such physical assets and qualities as strength, beauty and dignity were traditional loci of epideictic speech, and the goals of the genre were to praise the beautiful and blame the ugly (cf. Lausberg 1998, §239–40). Wichgreve's speech played with these conventions as well as with the traditional epideictic opposition between great and small, studying the subject's magnitude and amplifying its smallness and reminding us that by our choice of words we can magnify or diminish a thing.

Ancient rhetoricians like Aristotle and Cicero had noted that in order to praise or blame someone the method of renaming actions or a slight change in wording was very efficient; for example, we can say that someone has courage instead of saying that he is reckless or too daring. Wichgreve's defence was structured in the same way as serious praise. By abandoning the traditionally scornful names used for dwarfs, such as a pygmy, a small grain, a door handle and other expressions (*Nani, Pygmaei, portulae-ansae, salillum animae, homunciones, pusilli, moliones, parvuli pusiones, gradarii*) and by advocating the use of more neutral terms, Wichgreve created a favourable impression of dwarfs (p. 17).

Comparison of two persons or things was another important rhetorical device used here to construct an argument about the goodness of the subject. Comparison does not refer to a simile, but to a figure in which a comparison was made between equal or unequal objects, seeing an opposition, but also potentially a similarity between them.[3] Thus, shortness was here compared with colossal human beings, and shown to be equal to that quality or even better. In Wichgreve's view, short and tall people shared many qualities: they had the same functional body parts, the same physical structure, and they were born in the same way (pp. 15–17). But taking a universally accepted value of the excellence of magnitude as his starting point, Wichgreve demonstrated by examples (p. 27) that shortness in fact surpassed the commonly accepted ideal. He noted how small things were better than big ones in terms of usefulness, virtue, honour and beauty. For example, pearls and jewels were precious and valuable albeit small. Small bodies were beautiful compared with the colossal bodies of giants and Cyclopes. Small boats were more stable and firmer than big ships. Sharp weapons and swords were more efficient than those overlaid with gold. A short speech or book was often more persuasive than a long and verbose presentation. Wichgreve also cited historical witnesses and authorities from philosophical and sacred literature (Galen, Avicenna, Jerome) to substantiate his claims. Aristotle, for example, had argued that big animals had less courage than small ones, which were often powerful in being lethally poisonous. Large size was also presented here as being morally suspicious and identified with mere ostentation.

Another important device in praises was to compare the object to the paragons of the past, for example, an ordinary soldier was compared to the most famous war heroes in history (for example, Alexander the Great) and shown to exceed his famous predecessors in skill or valour. Aristotle emphasised that virtue was based on actions and deeds; therefore, in praising someone, an author should cite the person's actions as the products and indications of his good qualities. Honour came from heroic deeds in war, and victories in battle produced evidence of virtue and excellence. Thus, Wichgreve also celebrated small men's success and accomplishments in war and bravery in battle (pp. 29–39): David fought heroically against Goliath, and Titus Manlius defeated a Gaul who was double his size. Marcus Antonius loved small Sisyphus. Although an athlete, Milo died under a falling tree. Large-sized warriors also had great difficulties if they needed to jump quickly from the saddle, flee from battle or hide in a cave. Wichgreve assured his audience that dwarfs displayed the same virtues as great heroes and were superior to those who had more physical strength but less courage. Many emperors had relied on the wisdom of their small advisors, whereas according to Tacitus' description of the Germans, robust and tall men were often too open and sincere (p. 26).

Wichgreve mentioned historical examples of men who, despite their small size, had achieved leading positions in society as good emperors or otherwise represented moral or intellectual excellence (pp. 21–3). The list included such ancient leaders as the Spartan ruler and successful general Agesilaus, who was small, mean-looking and lame, and the famous names of Alexander the Great, Augustus, Caracalla, Diomedes, Menelaus and Ulysses. Later well-known figures of small-stature were St Paul, Philip Melanchthon, Erasmus of Rotterdam (whose name was commonly punned as *eras mus*) and Marcilio Ficino, who, in Wichgreve's estimation, was only half-sized. Many Roman poets like Horace and Cornelius Licinius Calvus were known for their small size, but also for their sublime, acute and nearly divine intellect. Physical reasons for this excellence were found in the circulation of blood that concentrated on a smaller area and accelerated all physical movements, including the movement of animal spirits from the heart to the head; this was the natural cause of the quick minds of small people. The discussion of virtuous, small size was further elaborated on by reminding of great Roman men who had lived in small houses (p. 19): Hercules had no need for temples; Caesar was born in a cottage; Romulus and Remus were brought up by a wolf and lived in a shepherd's hut; Cato lived modestly; Diogenes even lived in a tub; saints and monks had lived in caves, big philosophers in small gardens, and Jesus in a hovel. Smallness was linked with virtuous poverty and contrasted with the luxurious dwellings of notorious Roman emperors like Nero. Similar comparisons were made by Seneca in his *Epistulae* (66.3) and Petrarch in his *De remediis utriusque fortunae* and its dialogue on deformity and small size (II.1, *De deformitate corporis*), in which physical deformity was considered an unimportant gift of fortune.

Wichgreve's main arguments were that moral or intellectual virtue was the true basis of nobility and beauty, and the abilities and qualities of the mind were more important than physical strength. In the manner of Seneca (*Epistulae* 115.3; 66.4, *deformitas corporis, pulchritudo animi*) and Petrarch (II.1.36), Wichgreve stressed that a good man's soul could be tall, large, beautiful and great, even though the body was small (p. 19). Setting quality versus quantity and mind versus body, Wichgreve claimed that virtue did not exist in the stomach or on the face but – as the Roman satirists had already recognised – deep in the mind. By enumerating literary loci and authoritarian passages from Plato to Seneca, Wichgreve endeavoured to prove his argument that the human mind was superior to the body and human beings' animal side. Humans were always weaker than lions; peacocks rivalled men in magnificence, and a loud voice had been given to other animals as well as to men (p. 18). But the virtue of the mind belonged to men alone.[4]

Wichgreve's praise was here openly satirical when he emphasised the deceptive discrepancy between appearance (small size) and reality (inner wisdom). His pessimistic and satirical tone was also revealed in his dedication addressed to the university rector (pp. 8–10). In his words, in the early dawn the world had been crowded with Cyclopes but now it had lost a great deal of its strength, had become old and was losing virtue day by day. Since all things were expected to shrink in size before their final end, the same development was evident in his time, when men, who earlier had lived for hundreds of years, now hardly reached the age of one hundred. Smaller stature was one sign of the changing times. But this satirical perspective was then turned to parodical eulogy, as we have seen, whereby physical strength and size indicated less magnificent mental and moral qualities. It is difficult to know why Wichgreve decided to concentrate on dwarfs in his speech, but in addition to the joy taken in the playful arguments, there may also have been self-irony or other personal reasons involved. The praise is also continuously ironic and ambivalent in its estimation of small size, since when associated with such notorious emperors as Caracalla, it was hardly considered a sincerely positive sign.

Wichgreve's theme was rare but not unique, as already Petrarch's praise of small size in his *De remediis* has shown. Moreover, in his *Laus brevitatis* from 1649, Jesuit Théophile Raynaud (1583–1663) praised brevity in divine, human and natural beings. According to Isaac D'Israeli (1766–1848) and his *Curiosities of Literature,* Raynaud was "reading and writing through a life of eighty years, and giving only a quarter of an hour to his dinner, with a vigorous memory, and a whimsical taste for some singular subjects, he could not fail to accumulate a mass of knowledge which may still be useful for the curious" (1791–1823, Ch. "Secret history of authors who have ruined the booksellers"). D'Israeli recalled that Raynaud wrote 92 separate works, mainly theological and very often polemical – he was very zealous about souls, and he penned an extensive volume *Laus brevitatis, In praise of brevity.* In D'Israeli's words, in this book

> the maxims are brief, but the commentary long. One of the *natural* subjects treated on is that of *Noses:* he reviews a great number of noses, and, as usual, does not forget the Holy Virgin's. According to Raynaud, the nose of the Virgin Mary was long and aquiline, the mark of goodness and dignity; and as Jesus perfectly resembled his mother, he infers that he must have had such a nose.

Raynaud's book of several hundred pages ironically opened with a Horatian quotation, saying that he intends to be very brief in his treatment. He then dealt with the length of the Holy Scripture and enumerated Biblical examples related to length and shortness, advising that men's prayers and confessions should, with good reason, be long, but often penitence was as honestly expressed in a few words and perceived in a mere moment. In another section (3.IV), Raynaud concentrated on short bodies, claiming that small-sized men had more courage and spiritual strength than others. As examples of courageous minds, he mentioned Alexander the Great, Xanthippus the Spartan and St Paul, whose name already revealed his small stature, *paululus.* Small insects could show great virtue (industrious and beautiful bees and ants) or strength (poisonous scorpions). Raynaud did not forget the ears: they were also nicer when small, since large ears belonged to an ass.

These texts were concerned with the physically abnormal, but they did not simply ascribe moral or intellectual pretences to the body. The relationship between a man's physical appearance and his morals was not always construed in terms of unambiguous equivalence, and ugliness and vice did not always go hand in hand. Almost any physical feature could acquire moral qualities and be harnessed to serve moral criticism, as we have seen. But if physical dwarfishness was a moral quality, did this in fact call into question the very structures of such argumentation? Was there any reason to believe in the earlier satirical assumption of the revealing appearance, when in a clever rhetorician's hand every feature could be turned into a potentially significant symptom? Rhetorical satires were thus capable of breaking the normative views and moral stereotypes that were maintained by general satirical criticism.

Intellectual outlook and thinness in Jacob Balde's poetry

If lifestyle was believed to be reflected in a person's face and if general appearance acquired recognisable ethical qualities and indicators, then the obvious next question is what did a virtuous man look like? This, of course, depended on what virtue was understood to mean, but here the discussion centres especially on men who were dedicated to the contemplative life. One answer was given by Ulrich von Hutten in his dialogue *Febris secunda* in which he wrote that fever could produce in a man a trustworthy physical constitution that included the pallor and thinness associated with ardent studies. In Fever's words:

> First I will make you slim so that you become quick in your movements, because you have now acquired some weight and people may come to think that you are lazy and inefficient. Then I will give you a serious countenance to turn away all suspicion of frivolity, since there is surely something unpleasant in your excessive laughter and joking. (1860, p. 134)

The new look created for the author was one of Fever's several benefits, and here she appealed especially to the patient's proper intellectual features, which should indicate time spent at the desk. Hutten himself ironically responded that he only wished to please the women; he doubted whether they would be satisfied with a sick man's features.

A wise man's "sick" face had several of those pathological features that were mentioned, for example, in Laurent Joubert's medical treatise on quartan fever. There he argued that "it is a well known fact that sadness, fear and worries all have their impact not only on the mind, but also on the body, which turns cold and dry. The signs of this morbid condition are pallor or dark skin colour, thinness [...]" (1567, Caput IIII, p. 21.) In his influential French work on laughter, *Traité du ris* (1579), Joubert had also claimed that "those who give themselves completely to study and contemplation, or to some great enterprise, are almost all *agelasts*, sad, rude, severe, and have knitted brows, because the vital strength having been weakened by the consumption of spirits, they have little blood left, and that little is as coarse as the atrabilious kind" (1980, p. 104; trans. David de Rocher; cf. Kivistö 2008b).

A virtuous body and a face worthy of an intellectual were also discussed in Jacob Balde's satirical poetry. Balde praised thinness in his verse consolation, *Agathyrsus* (1638), and then later composed an ironic palinode and an apology for obesity, *Antagathyrsus sive apologia pinguium* (1658), giving both these characteristics moral interpretations. Balde himself was a devote ascetic, whose body was exceptionally skinny and ridiculed even by his friends. In Munich, he established a congregation for thin people and those wishing to lose weight, *Congregatio macilentorum*, whose members followed a strict diet and an ascetic lifestyle (Stroh 2004, pp. 209–40). Thinness was for Balde a genuine ideal related to his Christian and Stoic worldviews, but in praising thinness, he was also well aware of the tradition of mock encomium, and he positioned his poem in this satirical and paradoxical subgenre (Stroh 2004, p. 214). In praising thinness in *Agathyrsus*, Balde invoked Thinness (Macies) as his muse, the patroness of chastity and the guardian of sanity (Balde 1638, poem 67; Stroh 2004, p. 220). Elsewhere in his lyrics he called Thinness a sister of Galen and vivid sanity (Baier 2005, p. 246). Thinness, like the itch discussed in Chapter 3, was associated with poverty and not generally considered a physical ideal, but here its positive possibilities were developed to the full.

Balde's ideas about thinness should be read vis-à-vis the views presented by Plato and Seneca concerning the value of the body. In Plato's philosophy, man was seen as being dangerously infected by corporality, whereby the body and its physical desires stained the purity of the soul and disturbed its healthy balance with morbid alterations and disorders. One solution suggested to this problem was that the mind purified and disengaged itself of the body with the practice of the theoretical life. The purity of the soul was attained when man devoted himself to action with the mind only and detached himself from the demands of the body as far as possible. Catharsis in this sense, as defined in Plato's *Phaedo,* was a philosophical concept intended to free the mind of the contamination of the body (Laín Entralgo 1970, pp. 128–30). Likewise, Seneca rejoiced when he was old that only his body and vices had become senile, but his mind had remained strong; he was satisfied that it had only a slight connection with his body (*Epistulae* 26.2). This passage was quoted in the conclusion of Balde's *Agathyrsus*.

In his *Agathyrsus*, Balde expressed Platonic and Senecan contempt for the stomach, calling the body a prison for the soul (poem 1) and, in the manner of the Stoics, advising men to throw off the heavy burden under which they laboured like Atlas or mules (poem 3). One obvious way to escape the physical condition and separate it from the soul was to lose weight. When the physical world was an obstacle to eternity, thin bodies, also called shadows or praised as mere bones, had, in Balde's thinking, achieved a higher life as spiritual beings, since their souls were already partly freed from worldly bonds. Men who were meagre in body were closer to the next world and thus also very apt to practice the Christian life. Just as Erasmus had earlier praised kidney stones for teaching him how to die, Balde also playfully seemed to compare thinness with a philosophy that taught men how to die: when the thin had already lost so much of their body, they were freed from the fear of death, here called their friend. Moreover, the dead did not differ much from them in appearance, since both had the face of a dying person (poem 70). But in fat people, dying and losing one's strength was, of course, a much bigger and more troublesome process, and death appeared to their eyes like cruel Thyestes (poem 71). Thinness was interpreted here as an outer expression of a spiritual characteristic, which had learned to deny the physical impulses and the demands of the flesh, which stood for the vanity of the world. Balde openly thanked Fortuna for all his illnesses, since they had helped his soul to free itself from its bestial qualities (Stroh 2004, p. 216, n. 27).

In addition to praising thinness in *Agathyrsus* Balde also attacked sturdy people and reminded of the numerous diseases that made their lives troublesome, including "internal sand" and Sisyphus' uric stones (poem 11), lethargy (poem 12) and gout (poem 13). He compared a thick and round face with goitre and with the Juvenalian ulcer that was turgid and inflamed (poem 9, *vultus tumens rotundis, / an vultus est, an ulcus?*). Using an earlier commonplace, he also suggested that pallor was the colour of the sciences (poem 47). These claims were then backed up by references to the physical assets of several remarkable men of history, political leaders and literary authors. Diogenes, Seneca and Plato were mentioned as three virtuous thin men so powerful that even tyrants were afraid of them (poem 50). However, men who were guided by their desires, like Paris, Prince of Troy, must have been fat. Obesity affected the intellect and the morals; Balde called flesh the wet nurse of lust (poem 51).

Balde's satirical encomium opposed the Stoic to the Epicurean lifestyle; their different philosophies were concretely embodied in the outer appearance. The thin body resulted from the ascetic Stoic life devoted to intellectual activities, whereas the fat body signalled that the man had a taste for the condemnable delights of life. Precedence was, of course, given to thin and virtuous men (unless they were excessively ascetic), who withdrew from earthly pleasures, concentrated on contemplating the higher world and manifested these intellectual efforts in their outlooks. Eckart Schäfer (1976, p. 217) has noted that in playfully eulogising thin men, Balde imitated the ironic representation of the sour-faced and plain-living pseudo-Stoics in Horace's epistles (1.19.12–14) where Horace writes "if someone were to imitate Cato, going barefoot, / wearing a fierce, grim expression and a skimpy style / of toga, would he reproduce Cato's moral character" (trans. Niall Rudd). Among the poets, Virgil was an ideal ascetic, whereas Horace was an Epicurean who represented the opposite category, the man with the suspicious, glossy and greasy skin (Schäfer 1976, pp. 138–41; Balde 1658a, poem 50).

Balde's debt to Horace has been noted earlier, but I wish to emphasise that Seneca's role in these discussions was more notable; Balde was in many ways simply recomposing Senecan philosophical themes. For example, the equivalence between fat bodies and thin, dull minds was noted in Seneca's moral epistles (88.19, *corpora in sagina, animi in macie*), and Balde's *Agathyrsus* ended in excerpts and maxims taken from Seneca's epistles in which he condemned the body. These Senecan passages included exhortations to free the mind from its slavery to the body, since "virtue is held too cheap by the man who counts his body too dear" (14.2, trans. Richard M. Gummere; cf. 65.21). In order to see the inner face – the soul – and his true value, a man should be considered naked and, if possible, even asked to strip off his body (76.32; cf. 115.3, on the beauty of a good man's soul).

The human soul and its virtues are also contrasted with the physical strength of animals: Seneca deemed it futile to develop the muscles or broaden the shoulders, since it was impossible for a man to match a first-class bull in this respect; instead, man should "limit the flesh as much as possible" (*Epistulae* 15.2; trans. Richard M. Gummere). Seneca used concrete images in censuring vices that appealed to Balde the satirist. Thus, gluttony was discussed in terms of the belly, as with the satirists: Seneca compared a man dedicated to pleasures with a wine-strainer through whose bladder a thousand litres of wine have passed

(77.16), and he criticised the amount of work and effort wasted on one insatiable belly (95.24). In his *De vita beata* he announced that he was looking for the good in man, not the good in his belly, which was roomier in cattle and wild beasts (9.4).

Obesity was an indication of a life wasted in futile pleasures. In his *Solatium podagricorum*, Balde playfully described the gouty man Trimalchio's morbid appearance as follows:

> What a spectacle he gave to folk when waddling home from a meat market or drinking-bout! His inflated face with chubby cheeks competed with the wind and, as far as I know, his gusts and blowing often overcame it. What a prodigy, a man with a triple chin and a simple mind! Consider and measure his weight, if you can, weighing machine! [...] His stomach is bottomless, waist measurement is over ten feet, thighs grow daily in width, knee-joints nod, knees totter, and shanks swell, acquiring the size of Swiss milk pails. What a spectacle! (1661, question 31)

Balde's words scornfully pointed at the man's colossal and terrible body stuffed with fat-like cement and making the man a burden, even to himself. But in his ironic palinode, *Antagathyrsus*, Balde exercised his pen in praising fatness, which had served above as an image of the physical self. First, he claimed that during the golden age there was not a single thin person in the world, nor pallor, horror nor disease, but all men were nicely corpulent and healthy. The first slender men appeared in the silver age, and when times changed for the worse, their number increased. With them came hunger, thirst, black bile, hectic fever and other ailments (1658a, poem 4).

Balde's description of universal degeneration probably owed its origins to Seneca's epistle (95.15–17) which likewise noted that earlier, men had been sound and strong, but along with luxurious habits and over-nutrition came paleness, trembling, a repulsive thinness (from indigestion rather than from hunger), fevers and countless numbers of other morally disposed diseases. But Balde continued this idea of negative development by counting the emergence of the thin Stoics as a further sign of degeneration; the Stoics, with their bony and hunchbacked appearance, displaced the earlier, beautifully corpulent men. Balde wailed about the feeble bodies of the Stoics, their delicate fingers and half-sized faces, scorning them as mere monograms or lines of men rather than whole bodies (poem 6). Ancient deities and nymphs testified to the superiority of obesity, since they were always turgid and full-blooded, except the deities of the forest, Pan and the fauns, who were thin by reason of their libidinous character, which never let them rest. Virtue and beauty (represented by the full moon, for instance) was here linked with fatness, whereas vices and passions, poverty, anxiety, ambition and envy burdened the thin body with visible consequences (poems 10–12).

According to Balde's *Antagathyrsus*, thin people were oppressed by different diseases, such as fevers and cough. They had serious difficulties in finding enough cushions for comfortable sitting; the fat man carried his padding with him (poems 13–14). A thin man was a terror to boys and a bad omen for mothers (poem 15). Balde attributed to fat people the virtues of friendliness, good humour, reliability and upright and open character, which revealed at a glance that the man was devoted to eating. Thin men by contrast were often secretly insatiable and thus hypocrites (poems 19–21). They were also in many ways inhuman. They were inflexible, hard and unemotional, lacking feelings of love or grace and hardly ever showing sorrow. Whereas the fat man cried his heart out at funerals and lions were known to weep and the sunshine could melt ice, the thin man passed through sad situations untouched, with dry eyes, like a pumice (poems 25–6). Their faces were always wintry, as if covered by eternal frost (poem 28).

Balde thus playfully teased the Stoics about their unbending attitudes and ideals of apathy. Other differences between these two groups were found in their dreams. Even when sleeping, thin people were aggravated by their desires, worries and fears of such things as losing their harvest, friends or money, having nightmares about wolves chasing their cattle and of cows losing their offspring. The fat man's dreams were sweet and careless, filled with fat and happy cows, abundant crops and gigantic grapes (poem 29). A similar disparity was found in their inventions: fat people had discovered useful things like the plough, white paper, medicine and the magnet and gave names to the winds, but thin men had only invented things related to war and torture. The list given in poem 47 enumerated several imaginary war machines and other inventions that had brought only destruction.

These two stereotypic modes of living were also given their representative characters among the historical figures, scholars and religious men of Germany. Of the earlier intellectuals, Thomas of Aquinas was introduced in *Antagathyrsus* as a man with a bull's face and a voice whose mooing was heard around the world. He had a shining, white and fleshly face (poem 51). Cicero's size has been disputed, but apparently he was slim (poem 52). The sturdy German Luther and the slender

Frenchman Calvin were then contrasted by asking which was more immoral (poems 58–63) – it will be recalled, Balde was a Jesuit. Luther is called simply a swine, but in the manner of fat people, he openly confessed his sins with his appearance, without concealing his Calydonian snout or suppressing his goat smell. Calvin was assessed as being more decent, but arrogant in his virtuosity. A third figure, Melanchthon, was also brought into the discussion and described as mere bones, looking as though he had just fallen out of a halter. Balde thus used stereotypic physiognomy in his religious polemics, poking fun and finding fault in the religious leaders whose views differed from his own Jesuit judgements. He also ironically claimed that thinness was not always a sign of sanctity, even though people may have thought so, nor did pallor and wisdom necessarily go hand in hand.

In addition to thinness, which was often associated with intellectualism, Balde also discussed other features generally thought to reflect a learned mind. An original treatment of the intellectual face was found in his long satirical poem, *Vultuosae torvitatis encomium* (In praise of grim faces, 1658), where he discussed the great benefits of looking severe, threatening and even ugly. This poem was placed in the tradition of the paradoxical encomium. In his *De studio poetico*, a discussion of poetics that preceded his *Torvitas* and also a defence of satirical writing, Balde noted that to some men his encomium must have looked like a paradox, alien to common sense and just as strange as praises of outright deformity, vices or monsters (1658b, pp. 44–5). Here Balde also observed that philosophers and poets neglected their appearance and outward splendour. This was morally relevant, since satires maintained the idea of a meaningful contrast between the inner and the outer appearance. The magnificence of the internal face, as Balde called the human soul, was more important than a handsome figure. In his words, a neglected outlook and a face that recalled a cave or a beast's den suited wise men and poets, and there were only a few, rare men who were beautiful from the inside out.

The parallel with dwellings was used in his *Vultuosae torvitatis encomium* (1658c, poem 1) as well: ingenious minds usually did not live in great palaces but modestly, like the ultimate example of facial ugliness, the Cynic philosopher Diogenes, who lived in a tub. Poverty, virtue and ugliness again went hand in hand, as in the good old days when the statues of gods were simple and hewn from wood or as in an old man's face with its sagging skin that reminded one of a ploughed field, the eyes covered by lids like a loose tunic. As in these parallels, deformity often concealed wisdom, whereas delicate or attractive philosophers were abject creatures. Truly wise men were simply ugly: the Stoic Chrysippus had a huge and monstrous nose, and Aesop was known to have a hump more conspicuous than those of Arabian camels (poems 2–3). In one of his Saturnalian odes, Balde consoled a man called Luceius Budius the Stoic and stressed that in his wisdom he should prefer deformity to beauty, because deformity protected men from lust and other evils (*Silvarum libri* 5.8). Aesop, Thersites, Hipponax and Socrates were mentioned here as well.

The physical forms of the famous ancient philosophers bespoke their wisdom and virtue. In his *Torvitas* Balde went through different philosophical schools from the ancient Cynics to the Stoics and the Pythagoreans, assessing their representatives in terms of their facial and bodily impressions. As may be remembered, many of them had destroyed their eyes or were otherwise deformed. Socrates was, of course, famous for his satyr face, whereas Pythagoras' ugliness was related to his diet. He would not take so much as a bite of an animal, but followed a simple diet of lentils (*lens*), beans (*faba*) and peas (*pisum*); as Balde punned, Pythagoras was a triplex senator and esteemed over such noble Romans as Lentulus, Fabius or Piso (poem 5). To those who claimed that the Pythagoreans smelled bad due to their nourishment, Balde responded that it was the odour of erudition. Balde asked whether it was not better to have a brain than a nose, to have wisdom rather than to smell good.

Aristotle was identified as a man who, according to some opinions, was a dandy, fond of mirrors, golden rings and soft fabrics, but Balde argued that especially when studying the animals and natural history, Aristotle looked like a sordid haruspex, wandering around in dirty clothes among horses, moose, panthers, lions and other wild beasts (poem 10). Later intellectuals enjoyed a severe appearance as well, being horrible in the face but miraculous in doctrine and giving no attention to their looks but solely to their minds. Copernicus, for example, had a face such that the stars would have abhorred it if stars could only see (poem 12). His work as an astrologer was seen in the satirical context as virtuous as well, since it expressed man's love for celestial things and contempt for the mundane. Playing with the similarity of the words σωμα and σημα, the body and the tomb, Balde noted that Peter of Lombard looked like his tomb (poem 13). Duns Scotus had an unpleasant facial colour that resembled the greyness of ash or a rough, rustic hempen tunic. Some wise men had learned to endure pain and disease, and this patience was seen on their internal faces, which, after all such trials of several decades, had acquired a pious and placid countenance, like uric stones that were gradually polished and smoothed and acquired an even surface.

Their ugly faces revealed that they despised their bodies and were completely devoted to virtue.

After discussing the philosophers in his *Torvitas* Balde turned to the poets on whose faces inspiration had left its recognisable marks. Having once been touched by insane wisdom, a poet went through a facial change as though having weathered a mystic tempest. Balde mentioned several notable ancient poets who, at least in his estimation, had been severe-looking, including Ennius; Lucretius who advocated eating only sour herbs; Virgil, whose countenance reminded one of old rustic Rome rather than of the city; and Juvenal who was severe in multiple ways (poem 17). Ovid was an exception, a delicate lover, but Balde, playfully censuring Ovid's erotic poetry, wished that he had been ugly as well and thereby an author of different kinds of verses.

Not only were the poets severe-looking, but also the muses had been erroneously depicted as soft and graceful maidens, due to the incompetence of artists; in fact the muses were severe and chaste women who despised all delicacies (poem 18). Balde also mentioned ancient deities and oracles who had had ugly faces; the Sibyl, for example, had terrifying and distorted expressions on her face when giving prophecies (poem 20). The ancient examples were followed by Balde's contemporary figures, including Marten Schoock, who, in Balde's words, had a huge polyp on his nose, which made him a terrifying sight (poem 22). All the poets were praised on the grounds that although their faces were ugly, their verses were majestic and divine.

Thus, Balde argued in his *Torvitas* that a grim face was an advantage to intellectuals, since it showed that they were much wiser and happier if they looked ugly – as they usually did –, because they had probably devoted their lives to wisdom and learning. An ugly face protected them from many vices, like selfishness, self-love and sensual pleasures, and thus allowed them to search for true beauty. A grim face was not an obstacle to acquiring wisdom, but it favoured its pursuit. A grim face signalled a virtuous life and made such a life possible. Balde's long poem was again followed by prescriptions written by Seneca, Petrarch and the Jesuit Jeremias Drexel, who supposedly confirmed Balde's ideas. Seneca's prescriptions were composed of sentences taken from his moral epistles and pieced together. These included various statements about the vileness of the body, such as "limit the flesh as much as possible, and allow free play to the spirit" (15.2; trans. Richard M. Gummere) or "the frail body [...] is to be regarded as necessary rather than as important" (23.6; trans. Richard M. Gummere). Balde also quoted here passages from Petrarch's *De remediis*. In Balde's playful view, thin and severe-looking intellectuals had thus achieved the virtuous physical constitution that Stoic philosophers and Christian ascetics so eagerly recommended. Nevertheless, owing to the textual irony and exaggeration of ideal thinness, Stoics and other learned men hardly escaped satirical treatment. Thus, Balde's satirical poetry was truly paradoxical in leaving the final preference either for thinness, fatness or ugliness hanging in the air.

Strange student diseases

Learned discourses – dissertations, disputations and theses – offered ample material for parodical treatment with the intention to delight and amuse. Several pseudo-medical studies were devoted to strange diseases to which young male students especially were readily exposed. The *Facetiae facetiarum* of 1627 contains a scientific treatise on a contagion called *cochleatio* by pseudonymous authors Hasio Leflerus and Volucrinia Lepidus. The thesis was defended at the Faculty of Penetration in the presence of both genders, which already revealed the primary interests of the disputants. In the usual academic manner the thesis began by explaining the etymology of the word *cochleatio* and specifying the quality of the patients, *cochleatores*, in German *Lefflers*.[5] These were men who were as fond of licking virgins as the starving were of eating dumplings (§III). This addiction was a serious disease, because the patients did not themselves acknowledge their sickness. As is remembered from the philosophical discussions on the previous pages, ignorance and lack of proper self-knowledge were the most aggravating symptoms of the sick soul. After giving the definition, the authors drew attention to the ways the disease was caught; this discussion continued to have obvious sexual undertones, since the disease was said to spread by contagion "from eye to eye, from mouth to mouth, from tongue to tongue", and if the worst came to the worst, it adhered like a pestilence in the veins and abysses of the flesh (§V–VI). The sight of "a topping dame" was a common cause of symptoms, which were further exacerbated by sweet and tender words like "my pigeon" or "my hen" (§VII). These first signs were soon followed by stupefaction of the senses, blindness and deafness, so that a common frog was falsely taken to be Diana.

The most visible symptoms were diagnosed in the external body parts, and this was the mildest form of the disease, which occurred in the mouth and the tongue or in the outer veins. If the contagion found its way to the heart, then real danger threatened, since the disease could easily form a purulent ulcer inside, giving rise to morbid and complicated symptoms such as tumours and obstruction, which were potentially lethal (§XXIV–V). Further signs included large whites of the eyes, profound sighs, double rings on the fingers, and tremors of the central nervous system (§XLI). As in other quasi-scientific medical treatises, sexual undertones were barely concealed here, and the symptoms, developing from their first occurrence to the inveterate state, reflected the process of sexual attraction and gradual falling in love that in its final conclusion led to marriage, ironically likened here to the utmost weakness. The texts give considerable space to the description of the symptoms, which imitate medical discourse and are largely familiar from earlier satirical discussions, like frequent pallor, but these signs are now parodied and used merely for amusement, without any moralising intent. For example, the sight of a nude girl caused feverish rigour (*rigor febrilis*) and other severe symptoms (*Nugae venales*, p. 222). Diagnostic and therapeutic passages contained sexual jokes: a doctor should carefully investigate (*inspicere*) his female patient and study her body constitution; this is important in order to determine the proper dose of medicine and to avoid *hypercatharsis* (*Nugae venales*, p. 223).

Another strange disease called *hasibilitas* was discussed by the praeses Fabius Stenglecrus Leporinus and the respondent Lepidus Capito in their *Theses de Hasione et hasibili qualitate*. The treatise was also included in the anthologies *Nugae venales* and *Facetiae facetiarum*. Whereas satires usually advised men to suppress their bestial qualities and instincts in order to achieve humanity and the good life, this thesis described a sick condition in which these very qualities had become concretely visible and the rational mind was enthralled by bestial elements. The authors may well have had earlier famous satirical metamorphoses in mind – Apuleius and his parodical view of the Pythagorean doctrine of metempsychosis and texts in which men turned into asses (Wireker's *Speculum stultorum*, Rigault's *Funus parasiticum*, Wilhelm Holder's *Asinus avis* or others) – when composing the text.[6]

The thesis discussed a species that surpassed conventional biological taxonomies, a metamorphosed body or, in Aristotelian terms, a completely new species, *novum ens* (I.1). This creature was a combination of a man and a hare, scientifically named either *hominolepores, leporehomines, homines hasios* or *anthropodasypus* (I.2). Like *cochleatio* discussed above, the condition was understood as a disease (*morbus*), this time having its seat in the intellect and ensuing either from the superfluity or the privation of the white substance in the brain (I.4). Consequently, the animal spirits were confused, the balance of the humours was disturbed, and the heavy and light elements became mixed, creating an overall confusion of the humours in the brain, agglomerating in the stomach and also resulting in some conspicuous and vehement gestures of the limbs. How the disease spread was unknown, but it was considered an epidemic, with the infected being found in all countries of central Europe (I.5).

The authors diagnosed three different types of the disease, depending on its main seat and the severity of the symptoms. First, the disease could affect the spiritual faculty (I.7), and this type usually afflicted great, handsome and learned men or those who wished to resemble them closely. Their spirits were naturally on a high level, and they despised all lower things. Their attitude predisposed them to self-praise, pronunciation of sublime verses and sentences, speaking in tongues and writing poetry, so that they would be declared the great lights of their nation. Further signs of this contagion were arrogance, boasting and a highly ornamented style of dress. All this ensued from the high level of the spirits (I.9).

The second type of this disease resulted from an error in the bodily humours (I.10). This type was never found in sober men, but susceptibility to it increased with excessive drinking and gluttony, which moistened the brain. Four subspecies were defined according to the dominance of the respective bodily humour. In the case of excess blood, the disease manifested itself in outbursts of laughter and made the patient ridicule himself (I.11). If the primary cause was an excess of black bile, then the patient turned bad-tempered and unsocial, and he refused to react pleasantly to laughter or to participate in discussions (I.12). He did these things in order to leave an impression of intellectualism, as though he were busy with important or divine speculations. The third type originated in yellow bile, and the patient's reactions were even more severe: a single derisive word made him arm himself and evoked the strong desire to murder and slaughter (I.13). The fourth group of phlegmatic patients consisted of addicted drinkers, and it gradually led to frequent vomiting, diarrhoea and outspoken behaviours (I.14). Typical patients in this category were well-known fools such as Grobianus and Rulcius.

The third major variation after these four subtypes of the erring humours was situated in the elementary habits (I.15). Its milder signs were to be found in colourful and luxurious clothes bought abroad and in social gestures, such as kissing hands and dancing (I.18). Among the patients were found men such as Cornelius, Eulenspigelius, Papa de Calvo Monte, and Claus Stultus, all familiar from the literature of folly (I.22). The symptoms mentioned were frequent and loud laughter, running around, obscene gestures, dancing, rolling the eyes, long hair and an effeminate appearance (I.23).

The second thesis in the same treatise concentrated on describing the therapy for this disease. The therapy depended on the severity of the patient's condition and how widely the disease had affected the brain (II.8). It was also noted that sometimes the stupidity, as the disorder was explicitly diagnosed, was chronic and contracted by infection; occasionally, it received extra impetus from a deficient education (II.10). When the sick spirits ascended from the bowels to the patient's brain, the case was very difficult indeed. The patient himself rarely noticed anything except occasional headaches (obviously resulting from drinking), sudden belches or farts, all of which bespoke the forthcoming crisis (II.17–21). As can be expected, the prognosis was not good, and death was always imminent (II.27–8).

Old and well-known remedies were deemed useless and ineffective here, but some new medicaments were recommended. First, one should try remedies that dispelled stagnated humours or changed their constitution; these dispersives of diseased material included frequent bursts of laughter, jokes, beatings, vexations, tribulations, explosions and the like, all of which could be given in stronger or milder doses (II.30). Second, as purgatives, different violent acts were used: plucking hairs, grinding, whipping, deposition, knocking down, hanging by the nose, holding swine in front of the face, and some of the more imaginative forms of beating and causing bruises: *syncopizatio* (causing unconsciousness), *condylismi* (breaking fingers), *ciconisatio* (stork-peckings) and *apocoracismi* (crow-peckings), which were often needed in severe cases to avoid lobotomy (II.31). Among the fortifying drugs, the most efficient in deleting the crudity of digestion was very simple nourishment or a complete abstinence from food. Reproof, wise admonitions, hard work and duties in proper doses were always useful (II.32).

The therapy offered here consisted of both conventional didacticism and mere violence, which resembled the painful medical treatments in *Eccius dedolatus*. One historical background to the treatment was the so-called *depositio beani*, a violent initiation ritual that freshmen had to undergo at medieval German universities (see Füssel 2005). In Thomas W. Best's words, the initiation included harsh beating in which "the greenhorns, regarded as beasts, were symbolically altered to gentlemen ripe for academe" (1971, p. 21). Best also referred to a comic handbook of 1480 that included a grotesque description of such an event, where a new student Johannes (as the first-year-students were usually called) was treated like a medical patient, his goat horns were sawn off and fangs pulled out exactly the same way as in *Eccius dedolatus*. A similar violent deposition ritual was found in Christian Friedrich Prüschenk von Lindenhofen's university satire *Academicus somnians* (1720, pp. 15–16). As late as the turn of the eighteenth century, legal discussions noted that this kind of practical humour was allowed and no punishment by law was required (Kivistö 2008a). This tradition of academic violence was also discernible in these pseudo-scientific medical treatises.

Early modern humorous texts often dealt with new students and their initiation in terms of physiology, disease and therapy. The *Nugae venales* contains three quasi-scientific disputations by pseudonymous authors with the following titles: Onuparius Pallaeottus and Lucas de Penna's *Disputatio physiolistica, de jure et natura Pennalium* (Physiolistic disputation on the licence and nature of the Pennals); Vespasianus Curidemus and Zachaeus Pertinax's *Disputatio de Cornelio, et ejusdem natura, ac proprietate* (Disputation on Cornelius, his nature and characteristics); and Cornelius Cerastus Cornanus and Cariolinus Tevetius's *Themata medica, de beanorum, archibeanorum, beanulorum & cornutorum quorumque affectibus & curatione* (Medical themes on the affections and cure of the first-year students, arch-abcdarians, freshmen and greenhorns). The nouns *Pennales, Cornelius* and *beani* mentioned here were typical designations used for young (and foolish) students. Cornelius also referred to horns, which had their specific symbolism in this connection, as will be shown below.

In the first disputation on the Pennales, the patient under consideration was a brute and untamed animal or a monster and extremely rustic in his manners. The novice was here reduced to an ass and a simpleton, only recently released from his mother's arms and having as yet no capacity for conceiving of the subtleties of student life. The disputation gave physical notes by which to distinguish this newly-born species from a real student. Unlike his advanced colleagues, the Pennalis was stingy and always worried about money; even in a symposium he was counting the sips. He used syllogistic expressions; girls liked him; he was timid, arrogant and loquacious, but a good Latinist. A physiological detail marking him was erudition hanging from his nostrils and mouth like worms. The final remarks centred on the definition of the creature, calling him a loquacious, sarcastic, biting, voracious, thirsty, rapacious and niggardly man. The characteristics were partly ambivalent and not merely mocking (such as the favour with the girls). The disputation concentrated on physiology and did not elaborate on the object's sanitary condition or medical aspects; this task was taken up by the other two texts.

The disputation on Cornelius is interesting because it defined the new student in medical terms that referred to the sickness of the soul. According to the medical doctors' estimation, the state of Cornelianism was caused by the passions of the mind. The matter of the disease was found in the bodily fluids: the patient's radical humidity was on an exceptionally low level and his native temperature weak, resulting in a very dry and frigid spirit, which was black, sad, and rarely smiling – in a word, a monster more horrible than Homer's Polyphemus, Virgil's Fama, Ovid's giants or the Horatian Chimera. The condition could be helped by sleep, since one who sleeps does not sin. If this simple remedy was not strong enough, then more complicated mixtures could be tested. These remedies poked fun at old medical ideas about the balance of the bodily humours, and how the dry and cold soul could be brought into balance by means of wine as a hot liquid. Since the disease was caused by low temperature, the heat of the body was to be stimulated by a certain mixture of Malvasian wine, slices of bread, and, in difficult cases, increased by stronger spirits. Sacks of gold could be helpful as well, when changed into useful utensils in taverns. The author found it amazing that wise men like Theophrastus, Galen, Averroes, Vesalius and others had not discovered these extremely efficient remedies. Another excellent medicament was recommended, this one made of pure gold and a vivid and fruitful virgin, but it should not be enjoyed more than five times a day in order to avoid the reverse effect of atrophy.

Similar remedies mixing medical vocabulary with sexual innuendo were frequently encountered in contemporary literature. In *Epistolae obscurorum virorum* medical language created obscenity, when Doctor Brunellus (referring to the ass in Wireker's *Speculum stultorum*) gave instructions for treatment that consisted of a simple herb named Gyni, which was growing in moist places and had a rank odour. The patient was advised to grind the roots of the herb with the juice, to lie upon his belly for a full hour and to sweat profusely (I.33; Kivistö 2002, pp. 125–6). In *Nugae venales* a prescription offered to readers for their betterment advocated taking two handfuls of virgin breasts, press them strongly until there emerged a resurrection of the flesh, and after that to mix things with things to achieve a good state of perspiration (p. 323). And a conceptual study of the good wife, *Bonus mulier*, gave the following parodical recipe: "Twice a day one has to eat; twice a night to touch the instrument; twice a week the young should dance; twice a month the old should copulate."

The third scientific discussion in *Nugae venales*, entitled *Themata medica, de beanorum, archibeanorum, beanulorum & cornutorum quorumque affectibus & curatione*, was thoroughly medical, as though a medical doctor had written it. It concentrated on a previously unknown disease that had recently become more common but was still without an effective cure (§1). The author distinguished among three classes of patients, with different degrees of injury. In the mildest form of the disease (diagnosed as *Beanuli* or *Monocerotes*), one sharp and simple horn was produced on the forehead (§7). The second type (*Beani* or *Bicornes*) added another horn (§6), while the third type was the most serious and enduring (*Archibeani* or *Polycornes*): it caused several black, bad-smelling and huge horns (§5). The disease was thus easy to recognise, since it created a number of conspicuous excrescences on the patient's head.

The seat of the disease was in the brain. Among the predisposing causes, the dissertation mentioned the country air that the students had been breathing in their first years at school and a diet consisting of the meat of horned animals, asses, scholastic bread, putrid cheese, beans and other Pythagorean, leguminous plants (all of which were famously flatulent) (§9–10). Symptoms included extravagant movements, such as false steps, running, dancing and other motions accompanied by loud voices, and bacchanals, apparently characteristic features of student life (§11). The quality of sleep, loud snoring and other strange nocturnal voices were also indicative of the illness (§12). The excrement was to be inspected, since the patient's nourishment probably consisted of absorbed scholastic dust, which accumulated in his stomach and did not allow the digestion of better nourishment (§13). This resulted in different further symptoms and diseases, like frustrated love and asinine desperation. The illness was possibly hereditary, but the closest reason for it was poor education and the resulting thick vapours and smoke, which occupied the patient's brain and were very tenacious and difficult to expel (§14). This material solidified into a corneous substance and created the external horns.

The discussion then proceeded to other medical symptoms (§15), giving the normal list of pathological signs but exaggerating them by adding several attributes and thereby suggesting the severity of the sick condition. Thus, the patient's pulse was strong, vehement, quick, hard, full, frequent, irregular, beating two or more times the normal rate in a single moment, and skipping. The urine was thick, turbid, bloody, smelling of horny beasts of burden, reddish, greenish or blackish, foaming, and there were frogs, lizards, bats, scorpions and dragons floating in it. The diagnosis relied on the traditional phases of examination – feeling the pulse, tasting urine and attending to skin and eye colour. It also involved paying attention to the movements and fragrance of the bowels, a piercing look in the cyclopic eyes, the black colour and quadrangular form of the head, huge and protruding teeth, hare-like and deaf ears, and all kinds of symptoms that were familiar from earlier satires but here were more numerous and imaginary than in the earlier texts. The literary background of the symptoms was also noted in references to the patient's face, which reminded of the famous ugly jesters in earlier literature – Aesop, Thersites and the clever peasant Marcolf who was familiar from the *Dialogue of Solomon and Marcolf* (see Ziolkowski 2008). Moral signs were also listed (§16), and these included the gait of a stork (of which Erasmus had warned boys in his *De civilitate morum puerilium*) and loose clothes that revealed the patient's huge and protruding belly; the gait and the loose clothing had been famously condemned in the moralistic sense by Seneca when describing Maecenas, whose looseness of manners was reflected in his careless costume, the flowing tunic that was always untied (*Epistulae* 114.4). Animal voices released from the patient's mouth were also mentioned.

This long descriptive passage of the symptoms was then followed by a prognosis (§21–7) and suggestions for treatment. The inveterate form of Archibeani was incurable, but new patients could be helped before their twenty-first birthday. The text here contains several epitaphs of former patients who had perished after having suffered maximal pain caused by the putrefying horns and the worms in them (§23–7). The conventional three phases of therapy – diet, medication and surgery – were discussed next (§28–46). The authors advised taking notice of the air quality, which should be breathed in university towns if possible. The diet ought to be light and easy to digest, so that the meat of bears or dogs was served only three times a day. Drinks should consist of wine and beer, of course, including such labels as Junker, Guckguck, Klappit and Glatsch. If water was served, it should be boiled with mice tails, hare ears, an asinine ass and nails. Further operations included the already familiar violent beating with different instruments and the use of purgatives, the latter being made of the excrement of all household animals, bird droppings and various agricultural tools (§35). Special emetics that caused evacuations through the nostrils and so on had even more complicated ingredients, which included a horse's cranium, ruminating cows' intestines and other animal parts (§36). The treatment culminated in an operation on the horns, which were first softened in a medicament prepared from a bull's penis and always taken before dinner or several times a day (§39). This could be substituted with smith's hammers or by ten-feet-long logs, or, if necessary, the patient's head could be subjected to an anvil. In the most serious cases the surgeon was called to help remove the horns by using his saw (§40–2). The patient was first tied up so that he could not move. Then the skin was removed, the skull opened, and the horns were pulled up by the roots. The operation was completed with a hot iron to burn away the roots that were left and prevent them from recurring. Finally, the salt of wisdom was put into the patient's mouth to expel putrefying substances. This therapeutic passage was very similar to the one in *Eccius dedolatus*, including the same operations, but discussing them in a different, quasi-scientific form. After the operation the patient had to fast for 46 days, carefully covered by an asinine pelt (§44). The discussion ended in a warning that total recovery was not likely, but some preventive medicines were nevertheless recommended.

The horns that were the chief symptom here, reminded of the horns of the cuckold, which were one of the legendary physical afflictions often playfully discussed in early modern texts (Tomarken 1990, pp. 192–3). The horns often referred to the imaginary attributes of the husband of an unfaithful wife. They symbolised the deceived husband's foolishness and blindness, when he did not himself notice a situation that was clearly visible to everybody else, as were the horns on his head. The horns marked his impotence and weakness, but paradoxically they were also praised. Eulogies of horns went through different objects having horned attributes like the noble oxen, the moon and the horn of plenty. The authors listed illustrious horn-bearers and gods wearing such animal crowns and concentrated on the virtues and the beauty of horns as physical objects. Dionysus and his satyrs were also mentioned as having horns. Even though in paradoxical praises horns were a sign of nobility, Beroaldo's dialogue among the three brothers suggested that Dionysus' horns made concrete the pugnacious animal character of the drunken man (1648a, p. 159).

All in all, such pseudo-medical discussions borrowed their diagnostic terms and pathological symptoms from medical discourse and earlier satirical and moralistic literature. In the manner of satire and philosophy, they found fault especially in the patient's brain and his passions. Parodical effect was created by the use of these earlier discourses, their moral symptoms and medical language with its different phases of diagnostics and conventional forms of therapy. Special attention was given to sexual symptoms and all kinds of intumescences. Pallor, ulcers and other physical signs that had been morally significant and bespoke vices in earlier satirical literature were now also diagnosed and often complemented with more imaginative further signs. But the purpose of the descriptions of these complex and exaggerated diseases was no longer to censure the pathological condition, but rather to amuse the audience with learned references, parody and grotesque playfulness.

The art of farting

The sounds and odours of the bowels were, of course, such an important source of bodily humour in the early modern age that they cannot be overlooked here. These discussions parodied religious discourse that gave so prominent an emphasis to spirituality, but here the divine breath that inspired the authors was produced in the cavities of the body. Several pseudo-scientific theses were composed that concentrated especially on the different types of farts. *Discursus methodicus, de peditu,* for example, was addressed to medical doctors and philosophers in particular, and was found useful by theologians and other learned men as well. The discussion of farts was very popular indeed and reprinted in *Facetiae facetiarum* (1615, 1627) and Dornau's *Amphitheatrum*. The author relied on medical views of the healthiness of releasing the bowels, and on such Stoic opinions that maintained that belching and farting should be free.[7] In the playful definitions of the concept of farting, it was separated from belches, rumblings of the stomach and ventriloquism. Further divisions were made on the grounds of the loudness and tone of the fart, from simple and loud Priapic bombards (in German *Arschknollen*) and shy virginal whizzes (*Puellares* or *Jungfraufürzlein*) to moderate Aristotelian farts (*Medii* or *Bürgerlicher Schiss*). The authors discussed the tone of the voices in correlation to the structure of the backside and the diet, since flatulent dishes – onions, turnips, beans, peas, leguminous plants and other simple rustic nourishment recommended in the satiric tradition as virtuous and healthy – were extremely efficient in creating such fragrances. Farts were also classified according to the main nourishment, including such amusing types as *pisones*, created by eating peas, and *cicerones*, by vetches. The author also referred to the already familiar philosophical commonplace about the tribe living near the Nile cataracts; farts should never be so loud as to damage someone's hearing.

In this connection it suffices to note the repeated emphasis on the healthiness of farting, which prevented the gas from rising to the head and causing melancholy and insanity. Thus, farting playfully helped man to gain virtue that was so important to the satirists, since it kept a man's mind pure and free of bodily gases. Popular proverbs were also included in the discussion, such as the doctors' saying that "to defecate with farts was doing good to the internal parts" or "to evacuate without farting is as disappointing as travelling to Rome and not meeting the Pope". Rudolph Goclenius (1572–1621), a professor of medicine at Marburg, in his *Problemata de crepitu ventris* studied different vegetables that were efficient in creating farts, compared farting to music, answered the questions of why farts were often so odorous and why the Vandals farted frequently, made brief references to free farting in Stoic thinking and finally emphasised the naturalness of the phenomenon by comparing it to thunder and lightning (1619, pp. 349–54).

Very similar shorter discussions were included, for instance, in the *Nugae venales* (pp. 4–5). The importance of the theme was evident in the collection's opening – a cluster of short stories dealing with farts. For example, different occupations had their characteristic odours: the pharmacist's fart smelled of aromatic wine and anise; the jurist farted pure gold. Two anecdotes concentrated on the essence of the fart (pp. 8–9): it was considered substantial, since it was easily sensed, consisting of clear characteristics and having recognisable properties such as length, latitude and profundity – as may be remembered, these attributes also characterised the human soul in Wichgreve's speech on dwarfs and in Petrarch's *De remediis* (II.1.26). But the fart was also spiritual, for it was invisible, impossible to touch, yet heard and smelled. These discussions parodied medical views about the sense of smell and the substance of odours; Daniel Sennert, for example, argued that all odours were incorporeal (1628, p. 116, *De sensibus externis*). Philosophers, for their part, were interested in knowing what was good, and according to Cicero, good was something useful, beautiful and honest. Not surprisingly, in *Nugae venales* (pp. 13–14, 28–9) the fart was found useful on this basis, because it had taught men many arts: music, of course, but also astrology, when the ancients predicted rainy and dry weather by considering the sound of their farts, the art of war and especially of bombardment, and navigation in a head wind. The beauty and sweetness of farting were proved by its musicality and because it frequently made men laugh. It showed honesty in being useful and healthy, whereas keeping back a fart could be fatal. A parodical almanac – a form well known from Rabelais's writings and Bakhtin's studies – was also applied in *Nugae venales* (p. 41), stating self-evident facts such as that in the coming year the gluttons will suffer from gout, the healthy men will feel rather well and the country folk will have fluxes from eating plums. In these discussions of farting, the morally critical intentions were already blown away, as if by the slightest breeze.

Even though early modern satirical literature recognised a number of texts that were basically harsh attacks against vices and describing in detail the horrors of the sick body, aggravated by luxury and drinking, this is by no means the complete picture of a multifaceted genre. Already the satirical paradoxes and disease eulogies have shown that satirical criticism did not mean simple aggression, but its intertextual layers, recurring images and playfully philosophical issues were as important as the actual censuring of vices. This chapter has continued broadening the view of satires that dealt with moral issues with reference to their targets' health, physical appearance and bodily condition. By vividly describing moral failings as diseases but without any moralistic instruction, these texts also parodied the earlier satirical tradition and any strictly didactic and moralising views. Thus, these writings playfully reacted to the former moral criticism, reused traditional satirical images and called into question moral stereotypes that earlier satires had advocated as valuable or normative. However, the reason that I understand the texts studied here as satirical instead of being merely comical is that they never completely lost their touch with moral issues, virtues and vices. Instead, by using the devices of grotesque and humorous exaggeration, this criticism nearly turned from satire into parody. The texts studied could also be read as representing Menippean satire, which assumed various shapes in the Renaissance, including a learned treatise on a foolish topic. Menippean satire was a learned form that celebrated "the playfulness of the amateur and the seriousness of the scholar" (Blanchard 1995, p. 43). These words fully characterise the texts studied above.

6
Satire as Therapy

Analogismus equidem postremum locum inter alia Medici instrumenta habet, & magis quam experientia decipere potest. Interdum tamen ad eum necessario confugiendum, ubi scilicet nec ratione uti licet, atque illa, e quibus quid colligi debet, ignota & obstrusa sunt, nec experientia confirmari possunt, sed res plane nova est.

Analogy is the last tool the physician ought to use, and it is less reliable a source of knowledge than experience. However, at times we are forced to resort to it, namely, where reasoning fails or in such completely new cases where the causes of things are unknown and obscure and our experience does not shed enough light on the facts.

(Daniel Sennert, *Institutionum medicinae libri V*, p. 1069, *De indicatione*)

Horace's satires have often been called non-satirical, and Boethius's *Consolation* has usually been taken as a serious philosophical work.[1] The same conclusions could be made about some of the early modern texts studied here, but in their case, I would argue, the conclusions would be false. Consolatory discourse, essayistic pondering on the good life, disease and suffering, and paradoxical subversion of expectations and values may not qualify as satirical features in themselves, even though Menippean satire was very fond of paradoxes. Rather these texts have many obvious similarities with Seneca's and Cicero's philosophical discussions, which they often quote, and even with elegiac poetry, although they often turn the elegiac lamentation around and advocate refusing pain and laughing at the seriousness of suffering in order to recognise the benefits of physical illnesses.

In my view, however, the features mentioned above also characterised satirical writing, from Horace's *Sermones* and Persius' Stoic learning to the Neo-Latin disease eulogies. Considering the ethical nature and the themes examined in the previous discussions, it is possible to broaden our understanding of the genre. Satire is often restricted to aggressive derision and mockery, but not even verse satire is mere scorn at people's folly, avarice and luxury. It often discusses ethical themes by using a richer and more elaborate register of devices, allusions and attitudes than is possible in a direct attack or in simple moral instruction. Especially in satirical paradoxes and mock eulogies, which W. Scott Blanchard counted among the most important subgenres of Menippean satire in the Renaissance, we observe a return to the ethical and essayistic approach characteristic of Horace and Persius, in which critical humour was invested with the study of ethical issues, virtues and vices. Thus, the traditions of verse satire and Menippean satire are not completely separate, as they have sometimes been considered in modern research representing the Roman and Greek satirical traditions, respectively; rather, they shared a common concern for studying ethical issues. Humour can be found in many other genres as well, but when the ethical issues are playfully discussed and the vices described and blamed in vivid and concrete detail, we are witnessing a continuation of the tradition of the early Roman satirists.

Widening the idea of satirical criticism has meant that this discussion of medical satire has not concentrated on simple attacks against incompetent quacks, which were so common in all forms of graphic and literary satire. Consequently, the texts studied have not only described humorous, scatological therapies, but treatments that can be seen as playful and rhetorical versions of philosophical remedies. The focus has been on satirical therapy, which offered warning examples of immoral people who deterred men from vices and advised readers to pursue the good and virtuous life. Satirists diagnosed vices, endeavoured to prevent them and also to heal the patients. The therapy offered by satirical doctors took many forms, from painful attacks against vices and folly in *Eccius dedolatus* or in Frischlin's verse satires to consolation in suffering. They also offered prescriptions in the fashion of medical doctors well versed in philosophy, ordering dietary regulations and other forms of sober admonishment for better living.

The role of disease was ambivalent. Diseases and pathological symptoms, including pallor, internal ulcers, gout, blindness and so on, recurred in the texts studied as indices of a man' moral failure to the extent that they became commonplaces and topoi in the descriptions of an immoral man. These symptoms and diseases thus acquired lasting moral significance. But in addition to signalling vices, these same diseases – fever, gout, sleep and even drunkenness – also acquired salutary qualities and beneficial functions that in more serious discussions had belonged to philosophy or medicine. Whereas in philosophical literature the role of the physician belonged to the philosopher, here it belonged both to the satirist and to the illnesses, which were called both medical doctors and salutary remedies that improved a man's overall condition.

Physical diseases were defended on the grounds that they healed the mind, restored its vigour and improved the intellect by leaving men time to devote themselves to contemplation and reminding them of the true value of things. They had positive effects on men's morals, since when a man was chronically ill, he learned related virtues such as patience, modesty and humility. According to Petrarch, patience was a good remedy against all vices. Due to their physical illnesses or sensory disabilities, men were forced to keep a distance from worldly clamour and forcibly prevented from physical pleasures; consequently, their minds became free and virtuous. Satirists in their pessimism assumed that men would not deliberately choose virtue and true good; in their ignorance, they would not often let even the doctor (or the fever) in, which was the worst kind of sickness. But when ill, men were indeed compelled to wrestle with eternal questions instead of dedicating themselves to transitory pleasures.

Thus, illnesses created for a man a Boethian prison, an asylum or a place of exile in which to ponder what truly contributes to happiness and to distinguish true good from false. Illness, blindness, a prison, watching the world with an ass's eyes, from abroad or from outer space were common devices in satires to separate a man from the rest of the mad world and to give him distance and a superior perspective from which to study things more perceptively. Thereby, he was paradoxically closer to the real world that was so valuable to idealistic satire, religion and philosophy. The body that was often negatively depicted in satires as an obstacle to eternity and the seat of the vices thus also acquired positive qualities. In satires as well as in philosophy, internal good qualities were always more valuable than the gifts of Fortune, and disease eulogies reminded of this evaluation. Balde's praise of thinness even advised men to give up their sinful bodies completely. As the benefits of diseases and drunkenness, the goals familiar from the Stoic and other philosophical discussions of the good life were often mentioned: happiness and tranquillity of mind. Contrast between mind and body was important in these arguments; satirical wisdom was intended to improve the mind no less than philosophy, and diseases and disabilities helped in this process. But the elusiveness of the genre also prevents a reader from drawing final conclusions here. Although satirical instruction aligned itself thematically with philosophy, the satirical way of turning abstract vices into concrete images of ailing bodies was often deeply humorous, exaggerated and parodical. As such, satires often remained mere gestures of admonishment and parodies of philosophical instruction.

Even though none of these texts should be taken entirely seriously, I have also tried to appreciate the idea that early modern satirical and comical authors often expressed in the prefaces to their *facetiae* collections, namely, that under the frivolous surface of jesting, there may be hiding some useful and beneficial wisdom and serious arguments as well. As the author of the preface to the collection *Admiranda rerum admirabilium encomia* put it (pp. 3–6), the reader should not search the text for spiny academic questions, lawyers' or medical doctors' serious discussions about unsolvable or ambiguous cases, advice about how to run the state or how to manage one's life. Instead, the stated purpose of the collection was to evoke admiration, amusement and pleasure in reading. The playful but learned stories were meant to refresh the mind of the reader oppressed by his workload and worries. In the preface the author pointed out that human reason loved such intervals of joking and play. But in his words, under this playfulness a benevolent reader may find some moments and passages that are useful for achieving a better life, understanding the mysteries of nature or even contemplating philosophical doctrine. This play with serious issues has also been considered a characteristic of Menippean satire, which not only travestied serious works and ideas, but also played with them and often maintained a curious balance between seriousness and play.

In his moral epistles Seneca explained that analogy was an important way of acquiring the knowledge of virtue, since nature does not teach men directly. Instead of giving knowledge itself, she gives men the seeds of knowledge. In Seneca's words, the vision of virtue was acquired by comparing events that have occurred frequently, and the good was comprehended by this comparison and analogy. Seneca explained the concept with a medical analogy:

> We understood what bodily health was: and from this basis we deduced the existence of a certain mental health also. We knew, too, bodily strength, and from this basis we inferred the existence of

> mental sturdiness. Kindly deeds, humane deeds, brave deeds, had at times amazed us; so we began to admire them as if they were perfect. [...] And thus from such deeds we deduced the conception of some great good. (*Epistulae* 120.5; trans. Richard M. Gummere)

In the same way, the early modern poetics explained the goals of satire by referring to the medical analogy. The functions of satirical writing were analysed in terms of pathology, diagnosis and therapy familiar from medicine. But it is noteworthy that the medical images did not so much come from medical discourse, but rather from ancient philosophy and Stoic thinking in which the analogy between vices and diseases and wise words and medicine was common.

Among the ancient philosophers Seneca in particular had a remarkable role in the satires discussed here. After all, he was also a satirist and his *Apocolocyntosis* became an important model for Menippean satires in the Renaissance. But in this context he has played a major role as a moral philosopher. Satirical authors often borrowed his phrases and referred to his moral epistles in looking for arguments on resisting pain, enduring suffering and seeing diseases as images of the sick soul. His epistles and Cicero's *Tusculanae disputationes* offered words and ideas used in studying diseases of the mind and the therapy needed for their improvement. In this sense satires not only attacked vices but also offered playful advice for enduring difficult situations and even in finding many advantages in them. The relationship between satire and moral philosophy that was often brought out in early modern poetics was thus strong and substantial. The medical analogy was never a mere decorative device, but a pervasive theme both in early modern satires and in theoretical statements about the genre. But satire's relationship to moral instruction was not simple or merely parallel. In praising the grim faces and slim bodies of the Stoics, Balde also ridiculed them. This ambivalence was characteristic of the satirical way of discussing morals, and humour and laughter also undermined the serious thesis the author seemed to submit.

Appendix: The Anthologies Used in This Study

ADMIRANDA RERUM ADMIRABILIUM ENCOMIA, 1666

(The texts marked with an asterisk are also included in the *Dissertationum ludicrarum et amoenitatum scriptores varii*, 1638)

Erycius Puteanus, *Ovi encomium*

*Philip Melanchthon, *Laus formicae*

*Franciscus Scribanius, *Muscae encomium*

*Justus Lipsius, *Laus elephantis*

*Cuiusdam Itali, *Oratio funebris in picam*

Incerti Authoris, *M. Grunnii Corocottae Porcelli Testamentum*

*Caelius Calcagnini, *Encomium pulicis*

*Daniel Heinsius, *Laus pediculi*

Girolamo Cardano, *Podagrae encomium*

*Willibald Pirckheimer, *Apologia podagrae*

*Guilhelmus Menapius, *Encomium febris quartanae*

*Jacob Guther, *Tiresias seu caecitatis encomium*

Artur Johnston, *Laus senis*

*Erycius Puteanus, *Democritus, sive de risu dissertatio Saturnalis*

*Andreas Salernitanus, *Bellum grammaticale*

*Caspar Barlaeus, *Oratio de ente rationis*

*Caspar Barlaeus, *Nuptiae peripateticae*

Marcus Zuerius Boxhornius, *Allocutio nuptialis*

*M. Antonius Majoragius, *Luti encomium*

*Janus Dousa, *Laus umbrae*

*Jean Passerat, *Encomium asini*

Conrad Goddaeus, *Laus ululae*

Marten Schoock, *Surditatis encomium*

Marten Schoock, *Fumi encomium*

Mantissa, Itali cujusdam Authoris, *Oratio funebris in gallum Thessalae mulieris; Oratio funebris in felem Florae viduae; Oratio funebris in canem Leonteum*

CASPAR DORNAU, *AMPHITHEATRUM SAPIENTIAE SOCRATICAE IOCO-SERIAE*, Vol. 2, 1619

(Only the texts used in my study)

Aulus Gellius, *Noctes Atticae* (17.12, *Thersites et quartana*)

Ulrich von Hutten, *Febris prima et secunda*

Gulielmus Menapius Insulanus, *Encomium febris quartanae*

Erasmus of Rotterdam, *Podagrae et Calculi ex comparatione utriusque encomium*

Willibald Pirckheimer, *Podagrae laus*

Salomon Frenckell, *Podagra terrore abacta*

Jacobus Pontanus, *Morbidi duo, et laus Podagrae*

Girolamo Cardano, *Podagrae encomium*

Johann Carnarius Gandensis, *De podagrae laudibus oratio*

Jacobus Pontanus, *Podagrae hospitium conveniens*

Georgius Bartholdus Pontanus, *Triumphus Podagrae* (and shorter epigrams and poems)

Pantaleon Candidus, *De Aranea et Podagra*

Podagraegraphia, hoc est, Libellus consolatorius

M. Tullii Ciceronis Encomium caecitatis (in *Tusculanae disputationes*)

Johannes Vulteius (Jean Visagier), verse paraphrases of Cicero

Jean Passerat, *De caecitate*

Rodolphus Goclenius, *Problemata de crepitu ventris*

De peditu, ejusque speciebus, crepitu et visio

FACETIAE FACETIARUM, 1627 (Rostock)

Christophorus Fahrenhorstius Lubecensis, *De Bancorottorum pessimo atque horrendo scelere practico Dissertatio Politica*

Albertus Wichgrevius, *Oratio pro Μικανθρωποις sive Homullis*

Ioannes Barbatius, *Barbae Maiestas, hoc est, de Barbis Elegans, Brevis et Accurata Descriptio*

Antonius Hotomannus, *Jucundus et vere lectu dignus De Barba et Coma*

Georgius Nicolasius, *Methigraphia, sive Ebrietatis Descriptio, Effectus Eius, et Vitia Annexa*

Delineatio Summorum Capitum Lustitudinis Studenticae in nonnullis Academijs usitatae

Onuphrius Pallaeottus, Lucas De Penna, *Disputatio Physiolegistica, de Jure et Natura Pennalium*

Erasinus Liechbützer, Theopompus Innocentius Spuelwurm, *Discursus Theoreticopracticus Continens Naturam et Proprietatem Actionum Pennalium*

Johannes Qvistorpius, *Orationes duae*

Vespasianus Curidemus, Zachaeus Pertinax, *Disputatio De Cornelio et Eiusdem Natura ac Proprietate*

Ogravittus, Dacrio Chiplicus, *Materia Merè Magistralis: Multisciorum Studiosorum Magistrorumque Multivas Miserias Maleque Moratos magistrorum Musis merentium momos*

Catharina Florida Paphiensis, *Theses Inaugurales de Virginibus*

Cunradus Trentacinquius, Joachimus Eberartus Ab Hannow, *Bonus Mulier, sive Centuria Juridica Practica Quaestionum illustrium: De Mulieribus vel Uxoribus*

Hasio Leflerus Narragonensis, Volucrinia Lepida Stutzerensis, *Theses De Cochleatione Ejusque Venenosa Contagione, Et Multiplicibus Speciebus*

Georgius, Cunradi Filius, Rittershusius, *Jucunda De Osculis: Dissertatio historica, philologica*

Dionysius Bacchus, Blasius Multibibus, *Disputatio inauguralis Theoretico-Practica, Jus Potandi*

Calliphonus Stentor, Hugo Cüsonius Landaviensis, *Disputatio De Jubilatu*

Josephus Cornigerus, Cornutus, Bartholomaeus Alecthrochoras Baro et Dynasta in Frawenberg, Weiberbusch et Jungferndorff, *Dissertatio Theoretico-Practica De nobilissima et frequentissima Hanreitatum Materia*

Heinricus Christophorus a Griessheim, Victor Rabe, *Disputatio Feudalis De Cucurbitatione*

Bombardus Stevarzius Clarefortensis, Buldrianus Sclopetarius Blesensis, *Discursus Methodicus De Peditu, Ejusque Speciebus, Crepitu et Visio*

Fabius Stenglerus Leporinus, Lepidus Capito, *Theses De Hasione Et Hasibili Qualitate*

Matthaeus M. Czanakius, *Nobile Scabiei Encomium*

Gripholdus Knickknackius ex Floilandia, *Flöia Cortum Versicale, De Flois Swartibus*

Georgius Scribonius, *Consilium Nuptiale*

Concept einer Supplication An die Röm. Keys. May. unserm Allergnädigsten Herrn, von Allen Eheweibern in gemein, etc.

Wolgemuth Grünwein, *Ein Nagel Alter Orden Oder Nasse Bruderschafft dess Weingrünen Creutzes*

Bartholomaeus Stilvester Bocksbeutel, *Verbessertes und gantz neu ergangenes Ernstliches Mandat, Befelch und Landsordnung Hermanni Sartorii*

Bonifacius Sartorius, *Der Schneider Genug- und Sattsame Widerlegung,* etc.

Wundergeburt dess Alten HelGotts Lucifers

P. Ambrosius, *Ein Dutzet Artlicher Gleichnuss mit dem Jesuiter und Floh*

Hans Pumbsack

Poema vom Wurmschneiden, und dessen zugehörigen Sarsach und sehr scharpffen schneidendem Instrument

Newe und trewe Baurhaffte unnd immer Daurhaffte Practica, auch Bosserliche doch nicht verfürliche Prognostica, und Wetterbuch

Catharina Rosabella, *Der Jungengesellen Prob: Darinnen gründlichen unnd eygentlichen gelehret wird was der rechte ware Underscheid eines reinen unbefleckten Jungengesellen und jeglicher anderer Mansperson*

Bacchanalia

NUGAE VENALES, 1720

Theses de Hasione et Hasibili qualitate

Floia Cortum versicale de Flois Swartibus

Disputatio physiologistica, de jure et natura Pennalium

Disputatio de Cornelio et ejusdem natura, ac proprietate

Themata medica, Beanorum, Archibeanorum, Beanulorum et Cornutorum quorumcumque affectibus et curatione

Cornelia Carnivora, D. Kuckelbrion, *Theses inaugurales*

Prophetia mirabilis

Publius Porcius Poeta, *Pugna porcorum*

Crepundia poetica aucta

Canum cum catis certamen

Notes

1 Introduction: Medicine for the Sick Soul

1 All translations from Latin, except where otherwise indicated, are my own.

2 Stories based on the equivalence of a thing and its shadow are very old and frequently found, for example, in discussion of payments due. King Laelius was paid a debt with the shadow of cows instead of the cows themselves; the shadow of a purse was used in the same way in some stories. In German literature, Christoph Martin Wieland described the hiring of the shadow of an ass in the tale of Struthio and Anthrax in his narrative satire *Die Abderiten* (1774–80) (see Nauta 1931). The phrase was also mentioned in Plato's *Phaedrus* (260c). To quarrel over the shadow of an ass became a widespread proverbial phrase used in the sense of arguing about trivial issues. For the philosophy of the ass, see Ordine (1996). For ass eulogies, see Dornau (1619, pp. 493–503).

3 On writer's disease, see Ovid, *Tristia* (2.15, *insania morbo*); Gellius, *Noctes Atticae* (1.15.9, *morbus* [...] *loquendi*); Seneca, *Epistulae* (79.4, *morbo enim tuo daturus eras*). See Braund (1988, pp. 40, 211, n. 45). Braund (p. 42) also refers to the pallor of poets, a condition thought to derive from lucubration, lack of sun or homosexuality.

4 For medicine and literature in the Baroque age, see Engelhardt (1992). He notes (pp. 30–1, 50–1) that the popularity of medical metaphors was related to the philosophical and theological analogy of the microcosm reflecting the macrocosm that was still valid in the Baroque age.

5 For the development of anatomical investigation, see Porter (2001, pp. 154–62). For anatomy and Renaissance literature, see Sawday (1995).

6 On anatomy, see Frye (1973, pp. 308–14); Blanchard (1995, pp. 28–9; for Burton, see pp. 135–61). Burton's *Anatomy of Melancholy* studies diseases of the soul and the causes (including diet, bad air, education, idleness and different passions) and various cures of melancholic madness in particular. The book is clearly satirical in several ways, for example, when arguing that most men are mad. However, Burton's book is too extensive to be studied here in more detail.

7 See Aristophanes, *The Wasps* (650–1, on the intent of a comic poet to heal the inveterate disease in the state) and (1043, on purging). Cf. Freudenburg (1993, pp. 74, 77, 81, 89); Gowers (1993, p. 283).

8 Cf. Propertius, *Elegiae* (2.1.57–70).

9 For therapeutic rhetoric in Renaissance consolations, see McClure (1990); and in Seneca, see Ficca (2001).

10 The medical analogy between philosophy and medicine in Hellenistic philosophy has been widely studied; see Nussbaum (1996); Tieleman (2003, pp. 142–57, on Chrysippus); Long & Sedley (1987, #65). Plato mentioned diseases of the soul in *Timaeus* (86b) and *Gorgias* (477e–8c; 505a–b). For Plato, see Lloyd (2003, pp. 142–75); Vegetti (1995); Pisi (1983, p. 11); Laín Entralgo

(1970, pp. 127–37). For Aristotle's medical language, see Lloyd (2003, pp. 176–201); Jaeger (1957).

11 Cf. Cicero, *Tusc.* (3.4.9, *perturbationes animi morbos philosophi appellant*); (3.5.10, *sapientia sanitas sit animi*); (3.34.82, *philosophia, cum universam aegritudinem sustulit*); Sellars (2003, pp. 64–7); Erskine (1997).

12 Cicero argued (*Tusc.* 3.4.7) that passions such as pity or joy should not be called diseases but disorders (*perturbationes*). However, the term *morbus* is often used in connection with all disorders of the soul (3.4.9; 3.10.23). On the difference between the terms of disease (*morbus*), sickness (*aegrotatio*) and defect (*vitium*), see (4.13.28–9).

13 See Seneca, *Epistulae* (8.2, wise words work as medicine, effectively healing wounds); (15.1, a statement on philosophy's role in improving health); (50.9, even bitter philosophy feels sweet if the mind is strong); (78.5, *totius vitae remedium*). For Seneca's medical terms and metaphors, see Migliorini (1997, pp. 21–94). Health was a common topos in letter writing in general.

14 For Plutarch's interest in medicine, see Babbitt's introduction (1971) to Plutarch's dialogue "Advice about keeping well"; Scarborough (1969, pp. 137–9).

15 Cf. Pasch (1707, Caput III, §7): *Sane in multis inter satyram convenit & philosophiam, quae ut perfectio quaedam animi est, & quemadmodum Cicero loquitur, medicina; ita satyra quoque mentis morbo medetur, pellendo scilicet & auferendo ex intellectu ignorantiam, ex voluntate autem & appetitu malitiam.* Cf. Pagrot (1961, p. 24).

16 Cf. Schäfer (1992, pp. 56–66) who deals with a number of early seventeenth-century scholars – Thomas Farnaby, Isaac Casaubon, Friedrich Rappolt, Christian Thomasius, Daniel Georg Morhof and Georg Pasch – who all noted a close connection between satire and moral philosophy.

17 For Roman verse satirists' (often ironic) attitudes to different philosophical schools, see Colish (1985, pp. 159–224); Mayer (2005); Freudenburg (1993, pp. 8–21); Mendell (1920).

18 This passage is quoted in Latin in Schäfer (1992, p. 59); cf. Pagrot (1961, p. 105).

19 Pasch (1707) deals with literary genres – dialogues, examples, apologies, character studies, and aphorisms – that taught morals. The history of satire forms the Caput III in his book.

20 On Celtis and Vadian, see Schäfer (1976, pp. 27, 47–8, 50). Cf. Pagrot (1961, p. 107, on Eilhardus Lubinus's similar views); Landino (1486, *Proemium* II, where Roman satire equalled philosophy).

21 For Renaissance Menippean satire, see De Smet (1996); Blanchard (1995); Relihan (1996). De Smet (1996, pp. 23–56) discusses the Renaissance humanists' views of Menippean satire.

22 *The Greek Anthology* (11.112–26) and Martial's *Epigrams* (1.30, 47; 6.31; 9.96; 11.71, 74) included a number of poems providing evidence of fear and mistrust of physicians' incompetence in the use of remedies and tools. For satire on doctors, see Wootton (2006); Bowen (1998); Wagner (1993); Engelhardt (1992); Cousins (1982); Scarborough (1969, pp. 94–104); Holländer (1905). For a short example of doctors' Latin gibberish, see IJsewijn and Sacré (1998, p. 345).

23 Cf. Montanus (1529, *sat.* 2): *Qui plures occiderit, Ars stat in experientia*; and *Nugae venales* (p. 33): *Quinam sunt omnium liberrimi? Medici, & carnifices; quibus solis licet hominem impune occidere, & cum homicidium aliis capitale sit, illis etiam mercedem affert.*

24 Cf. Bebel (1931, III.18, *De medico, Georgius, abbas Zvifuldensis*), (III.24, *De doctore*), (III.78, *De rustico et medico*).

25 For Balde's attacks against doctors, see Notter (2005, pp. 181–2); Wiegand (1992); Classen (1976).

26 On *medicus amicus* in Seneca, see Flemming (2000, pp. 67–9); Pisi (1983). The ideal physician of Seneca was instructed equally in medicine and in philosophy (Scarborough 1969, pp. 27–8, 113–5).

27 Cf. Plutarch ("Superstition", *Moralia* 168C), where a superstitious sick man ejects the doctor from his house, since he thinks he is cursed. On Plutarch's attacks on superstition, see Scarborough (1969, pp. 137–9). On diseases as signs of divine will, see ibid. (pp. 15–25); Juvenal (13.229–32, physical feelings are taken as divine arrows). On philosophy vs. superstition, cf. Nussbaum (1996, p. 50).

28 However, Juvenal ascribed to fortune the random power to affect human life. He claimed that "if Fortune so pleases, you may rise from teacher to consul" (7.197; trans. Peter Green) and observed that Lady Luck will raise men to the summit of worldly success when she feels like joking (3.39–40). In Juvenal's ironic view, the potential success of people was not in their own hands or based on their merits and moral character, as it should be, but depended on higher and random powers, such as emperors. Seneca claimed in his *Consolatio ad Marciam* (10.6) that some things in life, such as health, were not entirely in our power, since capricious Fortune could maltreat us as she wished. But the wise man did not allow these fortuitous things to disturb his tranquillity and freedom.

29 Metaphors taken from the field of pathology have been applied in political usage from ancient Greece to Baroque Germany; see Healy 2001; Brock 2000; Kühlmann 1982; Hale 1971.

30 For Balde's poem, see Hartkamp (2005). For hydrophobia, see Balde (1661, poem 68).

31 Cf. a scholiast's note on Horace, *Epistulae* 1.2.52 in Botschuyver (1935, *ad loc.* p. 350): *omnis podagra insanabilis est;* and on 1.15.6 (in ibid. p. 373): *"Cessantem morbum" aut generaliter quemlibet vult intellegi, aut specialiter podagram, quae vix aut nunquam pellitur.*

32 Cf. Persius (1.104–5, *saliva / hoc natat in labris*); (2.33, *lustralibus* [...] *salivis*); (5.112, *salivam Mercurialem*, hunger for money); Juvenal (6.623) of the idiot Claudius (*longa manantia labra saliva*). Cf. Bramble (1974, pp. 130–1).

33 The phrase "nails to the earth a particle of the divine spirit" was explained by the scholiast as follows (Botschuyver 1935, *ad loc.*): *Definitio animae; quod dicit eam particulam divinae aurae esse, sic et Vergilius (Aen. VI, 743) aetherium sensum atque aurae simplicis ignem* [...]. *Dum ergo corpus crapula gravatur, anima etiam humo adfigitur, id est minus valet caelestia penetrare.*

34 On Persius' medical imagery and language, see Reckford (1998, 1962); Migliorini (1997); Bellandi (1988, pp. 35–9); Anderson (1982, pp. 173–8); Pasoli (1982); Scivoletto (1964); Spallici (1941); Lackenbacher (1937).

35 Havraeus (1627, p. 33) also warned not to trust appearances by composing a cento of well-known proverbs: *Fronti nulla fides* [...] / *Spina rosa tegitur: / latet & sub gramine (anguis) serpens. / Fallimur & gestu: multis simulatio vita est.*

36 Landino commented on this Horatian passage (2.1.62–4), saying that bad people often appeared spotless and immaculate, while being vicious inside (1486, *ad loc.*). A scholiast, however, interpreted this passage to mean that Lucilius attacked innocent people also and deprived them of honour (see Botschuyver 1935, *ad loc.*, p. 313): *non solum vitiosos, sed etiam innocentes ausus est carpere illorumque honorem detrahere, quo unusquisque incedebat nitidus in animo per ora vulgi.* The satirical act of exposing the pretensions that lay beneath the skin was expressed through sexual innuendo.

37 Horace, *Sermones* (2.1.64, *nitidus*); Persius (4.14, *decorus*); Horace, *Epistulae* (1.16.45, *introrsum turpem, speciosum pelle decora*).

38 On skin metaphors, see Bramble (1974, pp. 146–8, 153–4).

39 On dropsy, see Migliorini (1997, pp. 44–5); Scivoletto (1964, *ad loc.* Persius 3.63); Lackenbacher (1937, p. 136). Bellandi (1988, p. 37, n. 28) remarks that Persius often talked about dropsy in referring to diseases in general, apparently because it was directly traceable to indulgence. Cf. Horace, *Carmina* (2.2.13, *crescit indulgens sibi dirus hydrops*). Cf. Bouchet (1927, pp. 25–6).

40 Cf. Bellandi (1988, p. 133) who records here a reminiscence of the infernal scenes in Virgil's *Aeneid* (6.201, 240–1).

41 Cf. Claudian, *Eutr.* (2.11–13): *Ulcera possessis alte suffusa medullis / non leviore manu, ferro sanantur et igni* (quoted in Wöhrle 1991, p. 13). The last words of this clause have since become proverbial.

42 On the metaphor of wound in ancient literature, see Wöhrle (1991); Migliorini (1997, p. 152); Brock (2000, p. 25). Wöhrle discusses in more detail how wounds have been associated with diseases of the state (civil war, luxury) and with specific passions such as love-sickness (Dido), envy and anger. Cf. Lucretius, *De rerum natura* (4.1068–9); Nussbaum (1996, pp. 172, 259). For *vulnus* in Seneca, see Ficca (2001, pp. 166–9).

43 Cicero, *Tusc.* (2.16.38, a wounded veteran); (2.22.53, a brave soldier was operated upon without being bound); (2.24.58–9, brave men do not feel battle wounds). For military asceticism in cynicism, see Desmond (2006, p. 20). In Juvenal's satires, Republican veterans and war heroes were decorated by old scars as if by medals, but they belonged to a world long past of which only the scars remained (2.73). In another passage soldiers have suffered from multiple wounds in their wars against Pyrrhus and the Carthaginians but the reward they receive in compensation is absurdly small (14.164).

44 On ulcers or hidden ailments, see Seneca, *Epistulae* (53.5, 7; 98.15; 99.1; 101.12).

45 Moreover, the word "wound" carried sexual symbolism and referred to female genitalia. On the face, cf. Landino (1486, on Horace's satire 1.2): *Facies: Totius corporis figuram faciem vocamus: neque solum animati corporis sed inanimi.*

46 Cf. Rigault (1684, *ad loc.*): *hispida, hirta, & pilosa tua membra; durae setae, ut porcorum, per brachia & corpus tuum, promittunt Polyphemum aliquem & Herculeum, atrocem, invictum, gravem & severum animum, non mollem.* Cf. the famous Juvenalian laconism here, *perluces* (2.78), where a see-through dress

indicated transparent behaviour. On this satire, see Gold (1998); Walters (1998).

47 Persius (3.43, 85, 94 and 96, *pallere*); (1.26, *pallor senium*); (1.124, *cum sene palles*); (5.15, *pallentis radere mores*); (5.62, *nocturnis* [...] *impallescere chartis*); (5.80, *sub iudice palles*) and (5.184, *recutitaque sabbata palles*). See also Reckford (1962, p. 489, n. 2).

48 Whiteness does not connote clarity or purity here, in which case the word used would be *candidus*. André (1949, p. 26) quotes Servius' (*ad G.* III.82) clarifying definition: *Aliud est candidum esse, id est quadam nitenti luce perfusum, aliud album, quod pallori constat esse uicinum.*

49 Rigault (1684, *ad loc.*): *Mira malae conscientiae descriptio, qua rei ac conscii, modo frigore, modo calore alternis vicibus torquentur: illud fit propter metum, hoc ob pudorem; nam utrumque malae conscientiae inest.*

50 Cf. Scivoletto (1964, p. 64); André (1949, p. 77), with further references also to Cicero, *De inventione* (1.51, embarrassment); Propertius, *Elegiae* (3.14.20, pudency).

51 For the *facies Hippocratica*, see Sennert (1628, pp. 739–40, with reference to Hippocrates, 1. *Prognost. aph.* 5–7).

52 Dornau's compilation concentrates on Latin texts. For some German satirical texts on gout, see Hans Sachs's dialogue with the gods (1544), Jacob Ayrer's *Ein Fastnachsspiel aus dem Ritterordem des Podagrischen Fluss* (ca. 1600), and Georg Fleissner, *Ritterorden des podagrischen Fluss* (1594).

2 Medical Meta-language: Renaissance Commentaries and Poetics on the Healing Nature of Satire

1 For the medical imagery in satire in Renaissance poetics, see Deupmann (2002, pp. 84–153); Classen (1976); Brummack (1971, pp. 290–2, 304); Pagrot (1961, pp. 81–95). Deupmann notes how seventeenth-century ethical discussions also used medical language when dealing with sins and their cure.

2 For Minturno's poetics in general, see Hathaway (1962, *passim*); Weinberg (1961, pp. 737–43, 755–9); for the passage on satire, see Classen (1976, p. 97, n. 109); Pagrot (1961, pp. 74–6).

3 Pontanus's *Poeticae institutiones* was used as a schoolbook throughout Europe in the seventeenth century. According to his own words, Pontanus based his poetics on Aristotle, Plutarch, Horace, Scaliger, Viperano, Minturno, Robortello, Vida, Cicero and Quintilian. About Pontanus and Jesuit rhetoric, see Bauer (1986, pp. 243–318).

4 Boethius, *Philosophiae consolatio* (I.5.11, *nondum te validiora remedia contingunt*); (I.6.21, *firmioribus remediis nondum tempus est*); (II.1.7–8, sweet medicine of rhetoric); (II.3.3, *nondum morbi tui remedia, sed* [...] *doloris fomenta*); (III.1.2, *remedia paulo acriora*). According to Relihan (2007, p. 5), the harsh remedy refers to Socrates' cup of hemlock.

5 Landino (1486, cxvii); Pontanus (1594, pp. 172–3, *Artificium satyrae*). For the pill metaphor, see also Deupmann (2002, pp. 99–102); Schmitz (1972, pp. 39–40); Pagrot (1961, p. 53); Weinberg (1961, p. 23).

6 Cf. Sauer (2005); Wiegand (1992, p. 252).

7 The passage is quoted in Latin in Robathan and Cranz (1976, pp. 297–8). Cerutus wrote paraphrases of all three Roman satirists in the late 1580–90s.
8 For Vavasseur's ideas about Menippean satire, see De Smet (1996, pp. 53–5).
9 Cunaeus was a student of Heinsius and a renowned Hebraeist who, in 1611, became a professor of Latin at Leiden. His *Sardi venales* (1612) is a famous Menippean satire written against the degeneration of learning and the foolishness of conservative theologians.
10 For Rigault as a satirist, see De Smet (1996, pp. 117–50).
11 On Robortello and Italian Renaissance poetics, see Hathaway (1962, on catharsis, see pp. 205–300); Weinberg (1961, pp. 339–40, on the treatise *De satyra*).
12 For catharsis in comedy, see Taylor (1988); Bennett (1981a); in satire, see Deupmann (2002, pp. 107–17); Birney (1973); in literature in general, see Abdulla (1985). For comedy as the purgation of sadness through laughter, see Weinberg (1961, p. 28); or of troubles that disturb men's peace and tranquillity (like falling in love), see ibid. (p. 317).
13 The popular Renaissance conception that by relaxing the mind and dissipating stagnated humours in the body laughter improved the physical condition has been widely studied. For the therapeutic effects of laughter, see Schmitz (1972); Kivistö (2008b, with further references to laughter literature).
14 For Heinsius's work on tragedy, see Meter (1984, on tragic catharsis, see pp. 166–74 *et passim*); Sellin (1968, pp. 123–46).
15 Heinsius (1629a, p. 54): *Satyra est poësis, sine actionum serie, ad purgandos hominum animos inventa. in qua vitia humana, ignorantia, ac errores, tum quae ex utrisque proveniunt, in singulis, partim dramatico, partim simplici, partim mixto ex utroque genere dicendi, occulte ut plurimum ac figurate, perstringuntur; sicut humili ac familiari, ita acri partim ac dicaci, partim urbano ac iocoso constans sermone. quibus odium, indignatio movetur, aut risus.*
16 When dealing with tragic catharsis, Heinsius explained that *expiatio* was an Aristotelian and *purgatio* a Pythagorean concept that was also adopted by the later Platonists (1643, p. 10; Sellin 1968, p. 127). The *Oxford English Dictionary* says that expiation means "ceremonially purifying from guilt or pollution". In the Aristotelian uses of the word "catharsis", it had both the medical and the religious meanings. For catharsis in antiquity, see Laín Entralgo (1970, on Plato, p. 127ff.; on Aristotle, p. 182ff.). Cf. Golden (1973), who raised a third sense of the term, that is, clarification of intellectual understanding. Meter argues (1984, p. 166) that Minturno saw that by tragedy all detrimental emotions were driven from the soul, whereas Robortello maintained that the catharsis applied only to the emotions of pity and fear, and these were not completely abolished but only reduced to reasonable proportions. According to Hathaway (1962, p. 293), Minturno attached a cathartic function to epic as well, but refused it to melic poetry, comedy and satire.
17 Cf. Sellin (1968, pp. 164–77, on Heinsius's influence on Milton) and (pp. 178–99, on Dryden). For Heinsius's followers, see also Brummack (1971, pp. 304–6). Mueller (1966) emphasises Milton's debt to sixteenth-century Italian criticism and also argues (p. 145, n. 15) that Heinsius said nothing of catharsis that was not found in the Italian commentators, especially in Pietro Vettori's commentary of 1560. But I wish to point out that this is not true of satirical catharsis, on which Heinsius clearly elaborated in an original way.

18 Socratic philosophy and the Socratic method of questioning were linked to Roman satire in some Renaissance commentaries as well. In his very popular commentary on Persius, Johannes Murmellius noted Socratic features in Persius's satires, drawing special attention to the word *semipaganus* used by the poet in his preface. Murmellius argued that Persius wanted to avoid arrogance and conceal his true erudition, in contrast to his adversaries who, despite their seemingly witty and eloquent speech, were nothing but braggarts. (See Pagrot 1961, pp. 52–3.) This equalled the famous Socratic irony.

19 Envy was an inevitable concomitant of comical laughter in Plato's *Philebus* (see Bennett 1981a, p. 196). Envy was also discussed in terms of sickness (*morbus, dolor*). Nicolaus Perotti, in his late fifteenth-century (c. 1498–1500) translation of Basilius's speech *De invidia*, noted that others' success fed envy and inflicted wounds on people's chests. The gnawing pain aroused by envy burned deep inside the soul and was not cured by any doctor. See *Basilii oratio De invidia ex Graeco in Latinum conversa per Nicolaum Perotum* (Venetiae).

20 For Aristotle's ideas about indignation and envy, see Konstan (2006, pp. 111–28). Konstan interestingly notes (pp. 127–8) that nemesis was an old-fashioned and high-minded term already in Aristotle, who used it for divine displeasure at human immoderation.

21 The chapter was part of his paraphrase of Horace's *Ars poetica* in 1548. See Weinberg's edition (1970, pp. 638–9); Pagrot (1961, p. 67).

22 It was a common ancient view that the laughable lies in ugliness and deformity. See Taylor (1988, p. 324), with reference to Cicero's *De oratore* and Quintilian.

23 Robortello (1970, p. 502) also mentioned an ancient tribe called *Phaestii,* which, according to the testimony of Athenaeus had been educated since childhood and trained in joking to the extent that some of the members regarded their unending hilarity as a plague sent by the gods. Therefore, they attended the oracle of Apollo wishing in vain to recover their seriousness. See also Athenaeus, *Deipnosophistes* (6.261c–e). For Robortello, see also Pagrot (1961, pp. 67–8).

24 Mueller (1966, p. 146, n. 15) refers to Heinsius's use of the veteran image in his commentary on Aristotle's *Poetics.* Mueller considers the image an expression of Stoicism that shows the strong influence of Robortello's theory of habituation.

25 These arguments are found in Heinsius's notes to the *Ars poetica*, where he discussed satyr play and comedy (Meter 1984, p. 109). The negative rating of laughter was continued in his *De tragoediae constitutione.*

26 Taylor (1988) argues that comedies represent ridiculous stock types such as comic servants and tyrannical fathers, not murderers. In his words, there are no real social concerns, virtues or vices represented in comedy, but mere literary and stage stereotypes to which the audience reacted with detached emotions. Because of these mere stereotypes, comedies do not have important moral reference either. Cf. Sutton (1994, p. 76), who notes that comedy is traditionally populated with personifications of social authority. Satire has similar targets coming from high society, but instead of showing them as merely ridiculous, satire considered them morally depraved. However, Bennett (1981a) convincingly argues that the emotional range of comedy is

more complex than is often thought and includes many negative feelings and aggression. Cf. Aristotle who saw that hatred was felt towards certain types and classes of people such as thieves or informers (Konstan 2006, p. 186).

27 For these comic targets and emotions relieved by comedy, see, for example, Sutton (1994, p. 69 *et passim*); Bennett (1981a); Birney (1973, p. 9).

28 Heinsius emphasised the importance of the story (*fabula*) and action (*actio*) in arousing tragic emotions (1643, caput III *et passim*; Meter 1984, p. 170), but in the case of satire he saw that it was the characters who were important (Sellin 1968, p. 138).

29 Sutton (1994) prefers this definition of catharsis in general.

30 For Viperano's poetics, see Weinberg (1961, pp. 759–65). In the manner of Scaliger, Viperano also rejected Persius' satires as incomprehensible, the linguistic difficulty being a reason that they did not manage to affect people's mores and lives.

31 The scholiast said: *Radere: peritus mores obtrectare vitiosos scribendo satiram, et obiurgationis animadversione corrigere, ut medici dicuntur carnem de vulneribus putrem, dum ad vivum perveniant, quo facilius curent* (quoted in Latin in Bellandi 1988, p. 37, n. 29). The purified flesh (*carnem*, in accusative) was close to a purifying poem (*carmen*), a pun that the satirists and grammarians were likely to have noticed. On *urere* and *secare* used in the sense of (moral) vituperation, see Seneca, *Epistulae* (75.7); Cicero, *De officiis* (1.38.136, *sed ut ad urendum et secandum, sic et ad hoc genus castigandi raro invitique perveniemus*); Bellandi (1988, p. 39, n. 34); Bramble (1974, p. 36). For the verb *vulnerare* in medieval commentaries on Roman satire, see Kindermann (1978, pp. 60–3).

32 Murmellius noted in his commentary (1516, xiiii^{v}) that *praecordia* was the place of hilarity, a view that was often challenged by referring to the heart as the true seat of joy (Kivistö 2008b).

33 For satirical aggression and punishment, see also Deupmann (2002, satirical surgery is discussed on pp. 138–46).

34 Persius (1.126, *vaporata aure*); (5.63, *purgatas aures*); (5.86, *inquit Stoicus hic aurem mordaci lotus aceto*); (5.125, *decoctius audis*). For ear medicaments and decoctions, see Celsus' *De medicina* (6.7.1C and 5); Lackenbacher (1937, p. 139). On the metaphor of ears in Persius' satires, see Anderson (1982, pp. 174–8); Bramble (1974, pp. 26–7); Reckford (1962). Persius had several antecedents in using ear imagery: Horace exhorted the reader to philosophical study by referring to the healing effect through the ears (*Epistulae* 1.1.7; 1.8.16), and Seneca, Pliny and medical writers all had used the images of deafness, ears or their cleansing metaphorically in their texts (Reckford 1962, p. 478, n. 1).

35 For *Eccius dedolatus*, see Bowen (1998, pp. 89–91); Jillings (1995, p. 10); Könneker (1991, pp. 155–68); Best (1971). The Latin edition I have used is Berger (1931), the English is Best (1971); the Latin original is also printed in Böcking (1860).

36 Best also notes the influence of Seneca's *Hercules Oetaeus*, for example, lines 1218–78 (1971, p. 28, n. 2), and discusses other literary background to the play (such as Aristophanes' *Plutus*, Lucian's works). Bowen (1998, pp. 89–91) stressed that there are classical quotations and reminiscences on nearly every page. However, I wish to stress that there are also several reminiscences to medical images found in Roman satire.

37 Cf. Horace, *Epistulae* (1.19.18), where he claimed that imitators of virtue drink cumin to resemble learned men who acquired pallor from reading books at night.

3 Painfully Happy: Satirical Disease Eulogies and the Good Life

1 For the bodily etymology of the word "luxury", see Britannicus (1613b, p. 28): *Luxa membra e suis locis mota & soluta dicuntur, a quo luxuriosus in re familiari solutus, ut scribit Festus. Luxuria est igitur omnis morum solutio.*

2 For paradoxical encomia, see Pernot (1993, pp. 532–46); Tomarken (1990); Colie (1966); Geraldine (1964); Miller (1956); Pease (1926).

3 For Renaissance paradoxes, see Colie (1966).

4 Carnarius practiced medicine in Padua. Siraisi (2004, p. 201) notes that Carnarius delivered his speech as an introduction to his lectures on Avicenna's work on joint diseases. See also Tomarken (1990, pp. 64–5).

5 Johann Fischart translated Carnarius's and Pirckheimer's gout eulogies into German. This *Podagrammisch Trostbüchlein* (1577) was then retranslated into Latin as *Podagraegraphia*, with several additions to the original texts.

6 Pernot (1993, pp. 537–9) presents the ancient division between different eulogies: *endoxon* praises good and noble things; *adoxon*, something vile or bad like demons; *amphidoxon,* something ambivalent; and *paradoxon*, death, poverty and other extraordinary or indefensible things.

7 However, for Neo-Latin poems and satires on epidemic diseases such as the plague, see IJsewijn and Sacré (1998, pp. 59, 68). For Nathan Chytraeus's *Epistola satyrica contra pestem* (Rostock, 1587), see Kühlmann (1992). Chytraeus's poem is not eulogising but records the horrors of a society affected by the plague. Tomarken (1990, pp. 91–3) deals with two Italian eulogies of the plague written by Berni, calling him probably the only writer to have praised this terrifying pestilence. Berni's arguments in favour of the plague were that it made social life easier and peaceful for the non-sufferer, because there were fewer people on the streets or in the church. Moreover, the death from the plague was swift. According to Tomarken (p. 269, n. 30), most Renaissance works on the plague were medical and moralising.

8 For some examples, see Tomarken (1990, pp. 180–2). She notes (p. 261, n. 62) that, although there are numerous Neo-Latin works on venereal diseases, they were usually serious studies, not satires. Jillings (1995, pp. 9, 17, n. 49) notes that syphilis was used in satirical moral critique only in a small number of works. For Neo-Latin poems on syphilis and other medical issues, see IJsewijn and Sacré (1998, p. 346). Unfortunately, I have not had a chance to see the *Laus gonorrhoeae* (1712) by Lullius Hilarius.

9 For the cult of Febris, see Sallares 2002, pp. 50–3; *OCD* s.v. *Febris*; Roscher I.2, s.v. *Febris*; Valerius Maximus, *Factorum et dictorum memorabilium libri* (2.5.6, *Febrem autem ad minus nocendum templis colebant*); Augustine, *De civitate Dei* (3.25, *Romae etiam Febri, sicut Saluti, templum constitutum*).

10 Even though Fever was rare as a literary character, personification of an abstract concept was a common device in fable literature, Aristophanes' comedies and Lucian's satirical dialogues. For imitations of Lucian, see

Robinson (1979, p. 112); for Lucian's medical language, see Langholf 1996. In the manner of Persius' fifth satire, Augustinus personified the vices of avarice and luxury in his *Sermones* 86 and 164 (Fetkenheuer 2001, pp. 75–6). One of the most famous early modern personified diseases was Fracastoro's *Syphilis* (1530), who was introduced in his pastoral poem as a shepherd. For personifications of abstract nouns that denote emotions, forces or else, see Hamdorf (1964).

11 For these diagnostic passages in Lipsius's satire, see Blanchard (1995, pp. 82–3). For Lipsius's *Somnium* and Menippean dream-satire, see De Smet (1996, pp. 87–116).

12 Cf. Jillings (1995, pp. 7–8); Tomarken (1990, pp. 69–70, on Hutten), and (pp. 176–80, on fever eulogies in France); Robinson (1979, p. 112); Best (1969, pp. 41–2).

13 Cf. Best (1969, pp. 42–3, 72).

14 Cf. Best (1969, pp. 27, 57).

15 For Menapius, see also Tomarken (1990, pp. 70–1).

16 Quoted in Relihan (2007, p. 59).

17 In Dornau's edition, Pontanus's poem is followed by shorter epigrams dealing either with his poem, the theme of triumphant gout, or representing Gout as a grotesque figure. Tomarken (1990, p. 66) notes that Pontanus's narrative includes parodical allusions not only to royal triumphs, but also to several classical works, such as Virgil's epics, and in its dream structure allusions to medieval romance. Allegorical triumphs were popular in Renaissance art and literature; for the triumphs of Money and Poverty, see Hertel (1969, p. 99ff).

18 See also Porter and Rousseau (1998, pp. 29–30). The story of gout and the spider was also told by Petrarch and mentioned by Johann Fischart, among others (see Tomarken 1990, p. 260, n. 58).

19 De Meyere's poem *In podagram, Eius dolores acutissimos ac incurabiles esse* is printed in Mertz (1989, pp. 218–21). Machaon was Asclepius' son and the famous surgeon of the Greeks at Troy.

20 For the dialogue, see also Tomarken (1990, pp. 68–9), who remarks that a macabre competition in terms of suffering makes this work different from other disease eulogies. She also briefly discusses (p. 66) Johann Sommer's similar comparison of these two diseases in an early seventeenth-century mock-tragedy *Colicae et Podagrae tyrannus*.

21 For Seneca's concept of pain, see Edwards (1999); Wilson (1997).

22 However, in the Middle Stoa Panaetius maintained that virtue alone was not sufficient and even the wise man needed external good and health to reinforce virtue. Therefore, Horace ridiculed the virtuous wise man, saying that he is free, honoured, a king of kings, and healthy, too, unless he has a severe cold (*Epistulae* 1.1.106–8).

23 One popular theme in Renaissance elegy was the poet complaining about his sickness (*De se aegrotante*). Such (autobiographical) poems described the physical pains experienced by the poet, criticised vanity and man's groundless trust in his own powers only, and reminded one of the transitoriness of all created things. Unlike paradoxical eulogies, the tone was not eulogising but resigned, complaining of excruciations and isolation from friends, praying for improvement, or praising and thanking God after the recovery.

For this tradition, see Kühlmann (1992). Cf. the Hungarian poet Janus Pannonius's (1433–72) elegy 13 (*Conqueritur de aegrotationibus suis, in mense Martio 1466*), reprinted in Schnur (1967, pp. 316–21).

24 Engelhardt (1992, p. 38), with reference to Andreas Gryphius's *süss der Schmerz* and Petrarch's *dolendi voluptas*. For Petrarch's ideas about fortune and virtue, see Heitmann 1958.

25 Cf. Colie (1966, p. 462), with reference to Ortensio Lando's *Paradossi Cioè*, 1543. For Stoic paradoxes, see Ronnick (1991); for the Cynic paradoxes, see Desmond (2006).

26 *Podagraegraphia* (p. 245, quoting Paul): *per multas tribulationes oporteat nos pervenire ad regnum coelorum*, (p. 251, quoting Genesis 3): *In sudore vultus tui vesceris pane tuo*, and (Job 5): *homo nascitur ad laborem*. On dangerous leisure, see ibid. (p. 253).

27 Cf. Horace, *Sermones* 1.1.80–7; 2.3.145–7. Martial had satirical epigrams describing sick beds covered by scarlet bed-trappings (12.17) and illnesses displaying foolish wealth (2.16). Martial also criticised patients who had become addicted to honey, nuts and other tasty medicines prescribed for cough; prolonged cough was just code for gluttony (11.86). In yet another epigram a man got sick ten times a year and every time claimed congratulatory gifts (12.56). On the sick room and friendship, see Flemming (2000, p. 69).

28 For *vita activa* and *vita contemplativa*, see Vickers (1985).

29 Gout was interpreted in this way already by Petrarch, who in his letters praised gout for the opportunities it gave for moral and intellectual development. Cf. also his *De remediis utriusque fortunae* (II.84, *De podagra*). On Petrarch praising gout, see McClure (1990, p. 203, n. 9); Porter and Rousseau (1998, pp. 30–1).

30 On Boethius, see Relihan (2007). Imprisonment was defended by studying the concept of freedom, asking what constituted true freedom, and stressing the freedom of the spirit from the vanity of the world. Usually, the conclusion was that imprisonment was good for the soul, since the character was improved when behind bars; prisoners also often became religious, which was good for the church (Tomarken 1990, pp. 148–51).

31 For the twenty virtues of gout, see the list in Porter and Rousseau (1998, pp. 34–5).

32 Cf. Annibal de l'Ortigue's "le Delice des galleux" (1617) (mentioned in Tomarken 1990, p. 187), and Angelo Poliziano's *Sylva in scabiem* (1475/1477), a poem of around three hundred verses describing and lamenting the poet's disease.

33 According to Celsus, scabies was a roughening of the skin that had various forms (*De medicina* 5.28.16). Syphilis was then known as *scabies Gallica* until Hieronymus Fracastoro wrote his *Syphilis sive morbus Gallicus* in 1530 (IJsewijn and Sacré 1998, p. 346).

34 See also Laín Entralgo (1970, p. 133). For remarks about scratching and pleasure, see also Xenophon (*Memorabilia* 1.2.29–30), where desire is compared to the feelings of a pig, which loves to rub itself against stones.

35 Sennert (1628, p. 137) gives the following definition of disease: *Morbus est partium viventium corporis humani ad actiones naturales exercendas impotentia seu ineptitudo, ab earundem constitutione praeter naturam ortum habens.* Cf. ibid. (p. 10), where Sennert defines health as follows: *Sanitas est corporis*

humani eas, quae secundum naturam sunt, actiones exercendi potentia, a partium omnium naturali constitutione proveniens.

36 For the concept of *eutrapelia*, see Kivistö (2008a); Schmitz (1972).

4 Wonderfully Unaware: Sensory Disabilities, Contemplation and Consolation

1 For the history of the five senses, see Claren (2003); Nordenfalk (1985); Schleusener-Eichholz (1985, on blindness, see pp. 482–592); Vinge (1975).

2 Landino (1486, *ad loc.)* distinguished here, by reference to Martial, between three degrees of blindness: *lippus* meant aching eyes, *luscus* referred to a one-eyed person, and *caecus* could perceive nothing.

3 The edition of 1627 that I have consulted includes a preface written in 1625, the satires, and the author's biography. The Belgian Havraeus was born into a noble family, studied in Italy, spent his youth in France and was sent to a prison in Belgium in 1580 after having criticised the Catholic church. He lived for 74 years, mainly in France and in Belgium.

4 Cf. Pieters and Gosseye (2008, p. 179). They also discuss, by reference to Huygens's Dutch consolation, two central topics of the *caecitatis consolatio*: the opposition between looking inward and looking outward on the one hand and the opposition between the physical and the spiritual eyes on the other.

5 McClure observes (1990, p. 18) that Petrarch drew on several therapeutic discourses, including "the remedies of the love poet, the consolations of the philosopher, the admonitions of the priest, and the salves of the doctor". McClure also discusses other Renaissance consolatory manuals. For Petrarch's medical and ethical ideas, see Bergdolt (1992, on *Remediis*, see pp. 90–101).

6 These were Antonius' words to blind Didymus (cf. Petrarch, *De remediis* II.96). For the inner eye, see Schleusener-Eichholz 1985, pp. 953–1075.

7 For Boethius's use of pathological language in his *De consolatione philosophiae*, see *tumor* (I.5.12); *perturbationum morbus* (I.6.9); *morbus* (I.6.17, 19; II.3.3; III.7.2), *aegritudo* (II.1.2).

8 For blind philosophers, see also Cardano (1542, p. 112, on Didymus, Democritus, Asclepiades); Esser (1961, pp. 104–5, 124–5, 138).

9 Claren (2003, p. 309) mentions Georg Trinckhus's dissertation with a very similar title, *Dissertatiuncula de caecis sapientia ac eruditione claris, mirisque caecorum quorundam actionibus* (1672).

10 For medieval discussions of similar fallacies, see Schleusener-Eichholz (1985, pp. 84–5).

11 For *laudes inopiae*, see Desmond (2006); Meyer (1915); for Aristophanes and the later tradition of allegorical wealth and poverty, see Hertel (1969).

12 For similar unpleasant sights, see Ps.-Seneca, *De remediis fortuitorum* (12.1–2); Petrarch, *De remediis* (II.96, *De cecitate*).

13 For the name Scipio, Puteanus advises consulting Macrobius, *Saturnalia* 1, caput 6.

14 Several ancient men were known by this name, but Puteanus probably meant the Stoic Diodotus, whose name was often mentioned among the ancient blind men and who, according to Cicero (*Tusc.* 5.39.113), devoted himself to

philosophical study and had books read aloud to him day and night. Thus, he did not need eyes in his study.

15 A French humanist, Johannes Ravisius Textor listed famous blind men in his popular encyclopaedia called *Officina*, which included anecdotes and strange facts of every kind. His list was far more extensive than the one given here and included ancient mythical and historical characters who had been blind from birth or became blind later in their lives.

16 For Seneca's ideas about blindness, see Esser (1961, p. 125).

17 Puteanus (1609, pp. 41–2, quoting Cicero, *Ad familiares* 6.4): *in omnibus malis acerbius est videre quam audire*; and (6.1): *oculi augent dolorem*; (1609, pp. 45, 48, quoting Quintilian, *Declamationes* 1.6): *Vitiis enim nostris in animum per oculos via est*; and (2.9): *Caecus non irascitur, non odit, non concupiscit.*

18 For Thomas Hobbes echoes proved that sounds do not exist, but are merely subjective sensations (Rée 1999, p. 23). Cf. Sennert (1633, pp. 575–6), where he explains how echoes are formed.

19 These passages are carefully examined by Reckford (1962, pp. 479–82); see also Bramble (1974, pp. 26–7); Anderson (1982, pp. 174–7).

20 Cf. Persius (1.59, a mocking sign imitating ass's, that is, a fool's ears). For the image of the ass in Persius, see Anderson (1982, p. 176); Bramble (1974, pp. 27–8); Reckford (1962, p. 480). Cf. Martial, *Epigrammata* (6.39, long ears move like a donkey's ears); Horace, *Sermones* (1.9.20–1, on dropped ears). Note the pun on the poet's cognomen Flaccus, "droop-eared".

21 Sullivan (1978) claims that the implied reference to the ass's ears of King Midas contains a reference to Nero, but Sullivan does not agree with the funny explanation given by a scholiast that both Claudius and Nero would have had particularly long ears.

22 About Franck, see Kivistö (2007).

23 This commonplace was also given in Vincent of Beauvais's *Speculum morale* (see Vinge 1975, p. 67). For the topos of Ulysses being deaf to the Siren song, see Vredeveld (2001). Vredeveld shows how in Christian discourse the wax represented the Christian faith; the mast equalled faith, reason or moral virtue; the sirens were sinful pleasures, unbelief or heretical voices; and Ithaca meant the true homeland, heaven. To the church fathers, Ulysses represented a true Christian, whereas in Stoic thinking he was an exemplary wise man, who heard and recognised the siren song, but passed it by. In Christian polemics, the accusations of blindness and deafness were often directed against the heretics (cf. Schleusener-Eichholz 1985, p. 546). Cf. Juvenal (9.148–50) where Fortuna ironically stops her ears from hearing a poor man's small wishes.

24 Gaius Fimbria was an orator and consul ca. 104 BC. Cicero says (*Brutus* 129) that as children they used to read his orations, but later on they were scarcely to be met with. In *Brutus* (233) he noted that Fimbria was unable to maintain his character; he was immoderately vehement and resembled a madman (*insanus*) in speaking.

25 Vincent of Beauvais (and Petrarch) also cautioned against flattery, subversive speech and blasphemy. See his *Speculum morale* (Liber III, Dist. V, Pars I, col. 874Cff.); Vinge (1975, pp. 66–7).

26 Likewise, in his praise of monasticism *De contemptu mundi*, Erasmus persuaded his cousin to abandon the world – like Ulysses sealing the sailors' ears – and enter a monastery (Vredeveld 2001, p. 869).

27 The list of the diseases is given by Plutarch ("Whether the affections of the soul are worse than those of the body", *Moralia* 501A).
28 Cf. Seneca, *Epistulae* (53.5–8), which is taken by Reckford (1962, p. 489, n. 1) as a paraphrase and expansion of Persius' third satire.
29 In Roman satire insomnia was also ridiculed; men, worried about their riches, were never allowed to recover their breath through relaxation (Horace's satire 1.1; Juvenal 3.232–4).
30 Franck (1681, §4) mentions here, for example, Ovid's *Metamorphoses*; Statius's *Silvae* (5.4, *Somnus*), and such contemporary authorities as Antonio Gazio, *Florida corona sanitatis* (1491, c. 262–3); Beverovicius, *Theses sanitatis* (pars I, lib. 4, cap. 2); and Balthasar Bonifacius, *Historiarum ludicrarum libri* (17, c. 1). Also Dornau's compilation is given here as a source for sleep eulogies.
31 References are, for example, to Homer, *Odyssey* (9); *Iliad* (14.233); Nonnos, *Dionysiaca* (31.143); Valerius Flaccus, *Argonautica* (8.69, *somne omnipotens*).
32 This had taken place either in AD 250 or 447. The sources for the information include, for example, Paulus Diaconus's *Historia Langobardorum* (1.4). The story of the seven sleepers of Ephesus was also told, for example, by Gregorius of Tours in *Miraculorum in gloria martyrum* (cap. 94) and *Passio sanctorum martyrum septem dormientium apud Ephesum*.
33 Hegendorff was a pupil of Petrus Mosellanus and involved in the Lutheran movement from early on. He became Dr Juris in 1536 and professor of Roman law at Rostock in 1540. He also wrote a paraphrase of Persius. He died of the plague in 1540. (Robathan and Cranz 1976, p. 287.)
34 The poem is printed in condensed form in Mertz (1989, pp. 88–91). See also Janus Pannonius's elegy 12, *Ad somnum, cum dormire nesciret* (Schnur 1967, pp. 310–16).
35 Balde's poem is reprinted in Mertz (1989, pp. 124–9); Häussler (1978). Häussler discusses the theme of sleep in the work of three poets (Statius, Balde, Hölderlin), but also considers the history of insomnia and sleep.
36 For vices ensuing from drunkenness, see also Hessus (1515, B1r).
37 For the benefits of moderate drinking, see also Hessus (1515, B2r–B3r).
38 In addition to Hegendorff's text, Tomarken (1990, p. 54) discusses other sixteenth-century praises of drunkenness (Gerardus Bucoldianus's *Pro ebrietate oratio*, 1529, Robert Turner's *Oratio de laude ebrietatis*) as forming a popular subtype of vice eulogies. Turner's oration, written in the later sixteenth century, appears to be amusing in its positive description of the drunkard's appearance, his shiny nose and harmonious snoring.

5 Outlook and Virtue: Morally Symptomatic Physical Peculiarities

1 For some French examples, see Tomarken (1990, pp. 188–90).
2 See Tomarken (1990, pp. 192–7).
3 For comparison in epideictic oratory, see Lausberg (1998, §404, 1130); Hardison (1962, p. 31).
4 For similar animal comparisons in medieval literature, see Vinge (1975, pp. 47–58).

5 I am not certain if the term *cochleatio* refers to Johannes Cochlaeus, a theologian still mentioned in a positive sense in *Eccius dedolatus* (Best 1971, p. 37; Berger 1931, p. 71), but who later became a dedicated defender of Catholicism, which could easily have made him an object of humanist-minded satirical attacks. But the word *cochlea* was, of course, significant; it meant "snail".

6 For the Renaissance reception of Apuleius, see Gaisser (2008); Carver (2007); Blanchard (1995, pp. 22–3). In *Asinus avis* (Tübingen, 1587), a young man called Marcus Bömlerus wanted to become an eagle, but because of a ridiculous error he metamorphosed into another imaginary creature. On the proverb *Asinus avis* referring to a ridiculous omen, see Erasmus's *Adages* (2624).

7 According to Cicero, the Stoics maintained that farting and belching should be freely admitted (Cicero, *Ad familiares* 22; quoted in Marten Schoock's treatise *De sternutatione*, On sneezing). Petronius' Trimalchio also shared this view, remarking that it was unhealthy to hold it in (*Satyricon* 47.1–7).

6 Satire as Therapy

1 For Boethius, see Relihan (2007, p. 1).

Bibliography

Primary sources

Admiranda rerum admirabilium encomia, sive diserta & amoena Pallas disserens seria sub ludicra specie (Noviomagi Batavorum: Typis Reineri Smetii), 1666.

Anatome joco-seria conscientiae antiquae antiquatae & novae nudiustertius natae. Authore I. A. S. C. H., 1664.

Antidotum melancholiae joco serium: Inspice volve vale (Francofurti: apud Joann. Bencard), 1668.

Aristophanes (1963) *Plutus*, Aristophanes in three volumes, 3, trans. Benjamin Bickley Rogers (Cambridge, Mass.: Harvard University Press).

Aristotle (1947–) *Aristotle in twenty-three volumes* (Cambridge, Mass.: Harvard University Press).

Augustine (1983) *Confessiones*, Corpus Christianorum, Series Latina, 27 (Turnhout: Brepols).

Balde, Jacob (1660–) *Poemata*, http://www.uni-mannheim.de/mateo/camena/AUTBIO/balde.html (home page), accessed 1 December 2008. [Includes, for example, *Lyricorum libri IV, Silvarum libri IX, Agathyrsus* (1638), *Medicinae Gloria per satyras XXII* (1651), *Antagathyrsus sive apologia pinguium* (1658a), *Dissertatio praevia, de studio poetico* (1658b), *Vultuosae torvitatis encomium* (1658c), *Solatium podagricorum seu lusus satyricus* (1661), *De eclipsi solari* (1662), *Urania victrix* (1663).]

Balde, Jacob (1990) *Opera poetica omnia*, 4, Satyrica, Wilhelm Kühlmann and Hermann Wiegand (eds) Neudruck der Ausgabe München 1729, Texte der frühen Neuzeit, 1 (Frankfurt am Main: Keip).

Balde, Jacob (2003) *Urania victrix – Die siegreiche Urania*, Lutz Claren *et al.* (eds) (Tübingen: Max Niemeyer Verlag). [1663]

Barbae maiestas, hoc est, de barbis elegans, brevis et accurata descriptio, per M. Ioannem Barbatium Barbarum amatorem, 1614 (Francofurti: in off. Michaelis Fabri) in *Facetiae facetiarum* 1627.

Barclay, John (1973) *Euphormionis Lusinini Satyricon* (Nieuwkoop: B. de Graaf). [1605]

Bebel, Heinrich (1931) *Heinrich Bebels Facetien, drei Bücher*, Gustav Bebermeyer (ed.) (Leipzig: Verlag Karl W. Hiersemann). [1508–12]

Beroaldo, Filippo (1648a) *Quaestio quis inter scortatorem, aleatorem & ebriosum sit pessimus* in *Variorum auctorum practica artis amandi, et declamationes Philippi Beroaldi* (Lugduni Batavorum). [c. 1499]

Beroaldo, Filippo (1648b) *Declamatio, an orator sit philosopho & medico anteponendus* in *Variorum auctorum practica artis amandi, et declamationes Philippi Beroaldi* (Lugduni Batavorum). [c. 1497]

Boethius, Anicius Manlius Severinus (1957) *Philosophiae consolatio*, Ludovicus Bieler (ed.), Corpus Christianorum, Series Latina 94 (Turnholti: Typographi Brepols Editores Pontificii).

Bonus mulier, sive centuria juridica practica quaestionum illustrium: De mulieribus vel uxoribus in *Facetiae facetiarum* 1615.

Britannicus, Johannes (1613a) *Iunii Iuvenalis Satyrae sexdecim cum veteris scholiastae et Joannis Britannici commentariis* (Lutetiae). [1501]

Britannicus, Johannes (1613b) *Ioannis Britannici interpretatio Satyrarum Persii* in *Auli Persii Flacci Satyrae* (Lutetiae). [1481]

Burton, Robert (1821) *The Anatomy of Melancholy* [...] *by Democritus Junior.* London: J. Cuthell. [1621]

Candidus, Pantaleon (1619) *De aranea & podagra* in Dornau 1619, 2: 229.

Cardano, Girolamo (Hieronymus Cardanus) (1542) *De consolatione libri* (Venetiae).

Cardano, Girolamo (1559) *Medicinae encomium* in *Hieronymi Cardani Mediolanensis medici quaedam opuscula* (Basiliae).

Cardano, Girolamo (1619) *Podagrae encomium* in Dornau 1619, 2: 215–19; and *Admiranda rerum admirabilium encomia*, 148–70. [c. 1546]

Carnarius, Johannes (1619) *De podagrae laudibus oratio* in Dornau 1619, 2: 219–24. [1553]

Casaubon, Isaac (1605) *De Satyrica Graecorum poesi, & Romanorum Satira libri duo* (Parisiis: apud Ambrosium & Hieronymum Drovart).

Casaubon, Isaac (1780) *Auli Persii Flacci Satyrarum liber* (Mannhemii).

Celsus, Cornelius (1953) *De medicina*, 1–3, trans. W. G. Spencer (Cambridge, Mass.: Harvard University Press).

Cicero (1967) *De oratore*, Cicero in twenty-eight volumes, 3, trans. E. W. Sutton, H. Rackham (Cambridge, Mass.: Harvard University Press).

Cicero (1970) *De re publica*, Cicero in twenty-eight volumes, 16, trans. Clinton Walker Keyes (Cambridge, Mass.: Harvard University Press).

Cicero (*Tusc.*=) (1971) *Tusculan disputations*, Cicero in twenty-eight volumes, 18, trans. J. E. King (Cambridge, Mass.: Harvard University Press).

Codrus Urceus, Antonius (1506) *Satyrae* (Venetiis: Liechtensteyn), http://diglab.hab.de/inkunabeln/72-quod-2f-3/start.htm, accessed 1 November 2008.

Crusius, Martinus (1587) *De visu & caecitate oratio* (Tubingae: apud Alexandrum Hockium).

Cunaeus, Petrus (1620) *Sardi Venales* in *Quatuor clarissimorum virorum satyrae.* [1612]

Cunaeus, Petrus (1674a) *Oratio XI, In Horatium* in *Viri Cl. Petri Cunaei JC. Orationes argumenti varii* (Lipsiae), 211–32.

Cunaeus, Petrus (1674b) *Oratio XII, In Juvenalem* in *Viri Cl. Petri Cunaei JC. Orationes argumenti varii* (Lipsiae), 232–49.

Czanakius, Matthaeus M. (1627) *Nobile scabiei encomium ad nobilissimos scabianae reipublicae scabinos* in *Facetiae facetiarum* 1627.

Decoctio in Böcking 1860, 544–8.

Discursus methodicus de Peditu, ejusque speciebus, crepitu & visio, in theses digestus, Bombardus Stevarzius Clarefortensis, Buldrianus Sclopetarius Blesensis (pseudon.), Disputabuntur autem in aedibus divae Cloacinae, a summo mane ad noctem usque mediam (Clareforti: apud Stancarum Cepollam, sub signo Divi Blasii, 1596) in *Facetiae facetiarum* 1615, 1627; and Dornau 1619, 2: 355–9.

Disputatio de Cornelio, et ejusdem natura, ac proprietate, Vespasianus Curidemus, Zachaeus Pertinax Hierosolymitanus (pseudon.) in *Nugae venales*, 143–57.

Disputatio inauguralis Theoretica-Practica, Jus Potandi, [...] *in Academia Divae Potinae praesidente Dionysio Baccho symposiaste summo & antecessore praecellentissimo, in Collegio Hilaritatis, sympotis suis praestantissimis publice exponit*

Blasius Multibibus Utriusque vini & cerevisiae candidatus longe meritissimus (Oenozythopoli: ad signum oculorum rubricolorum) in *Facetiae facetiarum* 1615, 1627.

Disputatio physiologistica, de jure et natura Pennalium, Onuparius Pallaeottus, Lucas de Penna (pseudon.) in *Nugae venales,* 120–42; and *Facetiae facetiarum* 1615.

D'Israeli, Isaac (1791–1823) *Curiosities of literature,* http://www.spamula.net/col/, accessed 1 December 2008.

Dissertationes de laudibus et effectibus podagrae quas [...] *anonymus compatiens publice discutiendas proposuit suis confaederatis,* 1715, http://mcgovern.library.tmc.edu/data/www/html/collect/Gout/DLP1/Title1.htm, accessed 1 December 2008.

Dissertationum ludicrarum et amoenitatum scriptores varii (Lugduni Batavorum: apud Franciscos Hegerum & Hackium), 1638.

Dornau, Caspar (ed.) (1995 = 1619) *Amphitheatrum sapientiae Socraticae ioco-seriae,* 1–2, facsimile reprint of Hanau edition 1619, Robert Seidel (ed.) (Goldbach: Keip).

Dryden, John (1968) 'A discourse concerning the original and progress of satire' in George Watson (ed.) *Of Dramatic Poesy and Other Critical Essays,* 2 (London: Dent, Everyman's Library), 71–155. [1693]

Eckius dedolatus: a Reformation satire, Thomas W. Best (ed.) (Lexington: The University Press of Kentucky), 1971. [1520]

Eckius dedolatus in Berger 1931, 65–99; and Böcking 1860, 517–43. [Latin]

Eckius monachus in Böcking 1860, 549–52.

Epistolae obscurorum virorum (1978) Aloys Bömer (ed.) (Aalen: Scientia Verlag). [1515–17]

Erasmus of Rotterdam (1619) *Podagrae et calculi ex comparatione utriusque encomium* in Dornau 1619, 2: 202. [1525]

Erasmus of Rotterdam (1969–) *Opera omnia* (Amsterdam: North-Holland).

Facetiae facetiarum, hoc est, joco-seriorum fasciculus (novus), exhibens varia variorum autorum scripta, non tam lectu jucunda & jocosa, amoena & amanda, quam lectu vere digna & utilia, multisve moralibus ad mores seculi nostri accommodata, illustrata & adornata (Francofurti ad Moenum), 1615, 1627.

Farnaby, Thomas (1650) *D. Iunii Iuvenalis et Auli Persii Flacci Satyrae, cum annotationibus Th. Farnabii* (Amstelaedami: Typis Ioannis Blaev). [1612]

Franck von Franckenau, Georg (1722) *Satyrae medicae XX* (Lipsiae: apud Maur. Georg. Weidmann). [Includes, for example, *De auribus humanis mobilibus* (1676); *Quam diu dormiendum* (1681).]

Frischlin, Nicodemus (1568) *Oratio de dignitate et multiplici utilitate poeseos.*

Frischlin, Nicodemus (1607) *Satyrae octo adversus Iacobum Rabum, novitium Catholicum, Apostatam impiissimum, eiusque calumnias, quibus sinariores hoc tempore theologos plerosque insectatus est* (Gerae ad Elistrum: ex officina Spiessiana). [c. 1567–68]

Frischlin, Nicodemus (1609) *Nicodemi Frischlini, cum in Q. Horatii Flacci Venusini Epistolarum libros duos: tum A. Persii Flacci Volaterrani Satyras sex, eruditae & elegantes Paraphrases* (Francofurti ad Moenum: Typiis Nicolai Hoffmanni).

Frischlin, Nicodemus (1615) *In ebrietatem elegia* in *Facetiae facetiarum* 1615. Partly reprinted in Schnur 1967, 164–77. [c. 1601]

Gellius, Aulus (1960–1) *The Attic nights,* 1–3, John C. Rolfe (ed.) (Cambridge, Mass.: Harvard University Press).

Goclenius, Rodolphus (1619) *Problemata de crepitu ventris* in Dornau 1619, 2: 349–54.

The Greek Anthology, 4, trans. W. R. Paton (Cambridge, Mass.: Harvard University Press), 1979.

Guther, Jacob (1666) *Tiresias seu caecitatis encomium* in *Admiranda rerum admirabilium encomia,* 245–76; and *Dissertationes ludicrae,* 493–528. [1616]

Havraeus, Johannes (1627) *Arx virtutis sive de vera animi tranquillitate satyrae tres* (Antverpiae: ex officina Plantiniana).

Hegendorff, Christoph (1519) *Encomium somni* (Lipsiae: Schumannus).

Hegendorff, Christoph (1526/1529) *Declamatio in laudem ebrietatis, mire festiva* (Haganoae).

Heinsius, Daniel (1629a) *Qvintvs Horativs Flaccvs, accedunt nunc Danielis Heinsii De Satyra Horatiana libri duo* (Lugduni Batavorum: ex officina Elzeviriana).

Heinsius, Daniel (1629b) *Laus asini tertia parte auctior: cum aliis festivis opusculis* (Lugduni Batavorum: ex officina Elzeviriana).

Heinsius, Daniel (1643) *De tragoediae constitutione liber* (Lugduni Batavorum: ex officina Elseviriana). [1611]

Hessus, Helius Eobanus (1515) *De generibus ebriosorum et ebrietate vitanda* (Erfurt: Mathes Maler), http://www.uni-mannheim.de/mateo/camena/AUTBIO/hessus.html (home page), accessed 1 December 2008.

Hessus, Helius Eobanus (1537) *Podagrae ludus* (Mainz: Ivo Schoeffer), http://www.uni-mannheim.de/mateo/camena/AUTBIO/hessus.html (home page), accessed 1 December 2008.

Horace (1975) *Q. Horati Flacci opera,* Edward C. Wickham and H. W. Garrod (eds) (Oxford: Clarendon Press).

Horace (1987) *Satires and Epistles,* trans. Niall Rudd (London: Penguin Books).

Hutten, Ulrich von (1860) *Opera quae reperiri potuerunt omnia,* 4, Eduard Böcking (ed.) (Lipsiae: in aedibus Teubnerianis). [Includes, for example, *Febris prima* (1518), 27–42; *Fortuna* (1519), 77–100; *Febris secunda* (1519), 101–43; *Vadiscus* (1520), 145–268; *Inspicientes* (1520), 269–308; *Bulla vel Bullicida* (1520), 309–36.]

Jonston, Artur (1666) *Laus senis* in *Admiranda rerum admirabilium encomia,* 277.

Joubert, Laurent (1567) *De quartanae febris generatione tractatus* (Lugduni: apud Ioannem Frellonium).

Joubert, Laurent (1980) *Treatise on laughter (Traité du ris),* trans. David de Rocher (Alabama: The University of Alabama Press). [1579]

Jus potandi, see *Disputatio inauguralis.*

Juvenal (1974) *The sixteen satires,* trans. Peter Green (London: Penguin Books).

Juvenal (2006) Decimo Giunio Giovenale, *Satire,* Luca Canali (introduction), Ettore Barelli (ed.) (Milano: BUR).

Landino, Christoforo (1486) *Q. Horatius Flaccus, Opera* (Venetiis). [1482]

Lange, Christian (1688) *Miscellanea curiosa medica* in *Opera omnia* (Frankfurt am Main), 1–132. [1666]

Lauremberg, Johann (1684) *Satyra elegantissima* (Kiel: Reumann), http://digilab.hab.de/drucke/xb-6861/start.htm, accessed 1 December 2008. [c. 1630]

Lucian (1962) *Lexiphanes,* Lucian in eight volumes, 5, trans. A. M. Harmon (Cambridge, Mass.: Cambridge University Press), 291–327.

Lucian (1967) *Gout and the Swift-of-Foot,* Lucian in eight volumes, 8, trans. M. D. Macleod (Cambridge, Mass.: Harvard University Press), 319–77.

Lucilius (1967) in *Remains of old Latin,* 3, E. H. Warmington (ed.) (Cambridge, Mass.: Harvard University Press).

Lucretius Carus, T. (1975) *De rerum natura*, trans. W. H. D. Rouse (Cambridge, Mass.: Harvard University Press).

Mancinellus, Antonius and Jodocus Badius Ascensius (1515) *Decii Junii Juvenalis satyrae sexdecim*. [Mancinellus, 1492; Badius Ascensius, 1498]

Martial (1993) *Epigrams*, 1–3, D. R. Shackleton Bailey (ed.) (Cambridge, Mass.: Harvard University Press).

Martianus Capella (1969) *Martianus Capella,* Adolfus Dick (ed.) (Stuttgart: Teubner).

Melanchthon, Philip (1527) *Medicinae oratio in laudem artis medicae,* Vitenbergae habita (Haganoae).

Melanchthon, Philip (1846) *Liber de anima* in *Corpus reformatorum*, 13, Carolus Gottlieb Bretschneider (ed.) (Halis Saxonum: apud C. A. Schwetschke et filium). [1540]

Melander, Otho and Dionysius Melander (eds) (1617) *Iocorum atque seriorum, tum novorum, tum selectorum, atque imprimis memorabilium centuriae* (Francofurti: e libraria haeredum Palthenianorum officina, cura Hartmanni Palthenii, anno partus Virginei).

Menapius Insulanus, Gulielmus (1619) *Encomium febris quartanae* in Dornau 1619, 2: 183–91; *Admiranda rerum amirabiliun encomia*, 203–44; and *Dissertationum ludicrarum scriptores varii*, 445–91. [1542]

Minturno, Antonio Sebastiano (1970) *De poeta*, Poetiken des Cinquecento, 5 (München: Wilhelm Fink Verlag). [1559]

Molstetter, Philip (1593) *Laus caecitatis* (Moguntiae: ex officina Typographica Henrici Breem).

Montanus, Petrus (1529) *Satyrae* (Argentorati: apud Christianum Egenolphum).

Murmellius, Johannes (1516) *A. Persii Flacci Satyrae.*

Nicolasius, Georgius (1620) *Methigraphia, sive ebrietatis descriptio, effectus eius, et vitia annexa exhortationis syncerae-seriae loco, vulgari hac incompti sermonis lacinia, producta in publicum, et Lectori exhibita* (Friburgi Brisgoiae), in *Facetiae facetiarum* 1627.

Nugae venales, sive thesaurus ridendi & jocandi ad gravissimos severissimosque viros, patres melancholicorum conscriptos. Editio ultima auctior & correctior. Prostant apud Neminem, sed tamen Ubique, 1720.

Obsopoeus, Vincentius (1648) *De arte bibendi libri quatuor, et arte jocandi libri quatuor* (Lugduni Batavorum). [1525, 1536]

Ovid (2000) *Publio Ovidio Nasone Le metamorfosi*, 1–2, Gianpiero Rosati *et al.* (eds) (Milano: BUR).

Pasch, Georg (1707) *De variis modis moralia tradendi* (Kiloni: sumptibus Joh. Sebast. Riechelii).

Passerat, Jean (1619) *De caecitate oratio* in Dornau 1619, 2: 262–4; and Puteanus 1609, 105ff. [1597]

Persius Flaccus, A. (1964) *Saturae,* Nino Scivoletto (ed.) (Firenze: "La nuova Italia" editrice).

Persius (1987) *Satires,* trans. Niall Rudd (London: Penguin Books).

Pétrarque (2002) *Les remèdes aux deux fortunes: De remediis utriusque fortunae,* 1–2, Christophe Carraud (ed.) (Grenoble: Éditions Jérôme Millon). [1354–66]

Petronius (1969), *Satyricon*, trans Michael Heseltine, E. H. Warmington (Cambridge, Mass.: Harvard University Press).

Pirckheimer, Willibald (2002) *Apologia seu Podagrae laus*, Ulrich Winter (ed.) (Heidelberg: Universitätsverlag C. Winter). (Also in *Admiranda rerum admirabilium encomia*, 170–203; and *Dissertationum ludicrarum scriptores varii*, 1–39.) [1522]

Plato (1960–) *Plato in twelve volumes* (Cambridge, Mass.: Harvard University Press).

Plutarch (1960–) *Plutarch's Moralia in sixteen volumes*, Frank Cole Babbitt *et al.* (eds) (Cambridge, Mass.: Harvard University Press).

Podagraegraphia, hoc est, Libellus consolatorius, duos sermones defensoriales in Dornau 1619, 2: 229ff.

Poliziano, Angelo (1613) *In Persium praelectio* in *Auli Persii Flacci Satyrae* (Lutetiae). [1484–85]

Pontanus, Georgius Bartholdus (1619) *Triumphus Podagrae* in Dornau 1619, 2: 224–7. [1605]

Pontanus, Jacobus (1594) *Poeticarum institutionum libri tres* (Ingolstadii: ex typographia Davidis Sartorii).

Pontanus, Jacobus (1619a) *Podagrae hospitium* in Dornau 1619, 2: 224.

Pontanus, Jacobus (1619b) *Morbidi duo, & laus Podagrae* in Dornau 1619, 2: 214–15.

Pontanus, Ioannis Iovianus (1954) *De sermone libri sex*, S. Lupi, A. Risicato (eds) (Lucani: in aedibus thesauri mundi). [1499]

Prüschenk von Lindenhofen, Christian Friedrich (1720) *Lepidi Philalethis Sannionis Utopiensis Academicus somnians, satyra in laudem modernae eruditionis conscripta*. In Parnasso Simon Rinobasilius Typotheta Phoebeus. [1659]

Puteanus, Erycius (1609) *Caecitatis consolatio* (Lovanii: in officina Typographica Gerardi Rivii).

Quatuor clarissimorum virorum satyrae (Lugduni Batavorum: ex officina Marciana), 1620. [Includes: Rigault's *Funus parasiticum*; Justus Lipsius's *Somnium*, Cunaeus's *Sardi venales* and Cunaeus's Latin translation of Julian's *Caesares*].

Quintilianus, M. Fabius (1970) *Institutionis oratoriae libri duodecim*, 1–2, M. Winterbottom (ed.) (Oxford: Clarendon Press).

Rappolt, Friedrich (1675) *Commentarius in Q. Horatii Flacci Satyras & Epistolas omnes* (Lipsiae: sumptibus Joh. Grossii & Soc., Literis Christophori Uhmanni).

Ravisius Textor, Joannes (1595) *Theatrum poeticum et historicum, sive Officina* (Basiliae).

Raynaud, Theophilè (1649) *Laus brevitatis, per dictyaca de brevitate et longitudine in divinis, humanis, et naturalibus* (Gratianopoli: apud Petrum Fremon).

Rigault, Nicolas (1620) *Funus parasiticum* in *Quatuor clarissimorum virorum satyrae*. [1599]

Rigault, Nicolas (1684) *De satira Juvenalis* in *D. Junii Juvenalis & Auli Persii Flacci Satyrae cum veteris scholiastae & variorum commentariis, editio nova* (Amstelaedami: apud Henricum Wetstenium). [c. 1616]

Robortello, Francesco (1970) *Explicatio eorum omnium quae ad satyram pertinent* in Bernard Weinberg (ed.) *Trattati di poetica e retorica del cinquecento*, I (Bari: Gius. Laterza & Figli), 495–507. [1548]

Scaliger, Iulius Caesar (1994–5) *Poetices libri septem*, vols 1 and 3, Luc Deitz (ed.) (Stuttgart–Bad Cannstatt). [1561]

Schoock, Marten (1664) *De sternutatione tractatus copiosus*, 2 ed. (Amstelodami: apud Petrum van den Berge).

Schoock, Marten (1666) *Surditatis encomium* in *Admiranda rerum admirabilium encomia*, 602–25.
Seneca (1967, 1989, 1996) *Ad Lucilium epistulae morales*, 1–3, trans. Richard M. Gummere (Cambridge, Mass.: Harvard University Press).
Seneca (1969) *Apocolocyntosis*, trans. W. H. D. Rouse (Cambridge, Mass.: Harvard University Press).
Seneca (1996) *Moral essays*, trans. John W. Basore (Cambridge, Mass.: Harvard University Press).
Sennert, Daniel (1628) *Institutionum medicinae libri V* (Wittebergae: apud haeredes Zach. Schüreri Sen.).
Sennert, Daniel (1633) *Epitome naturalis scientiae* (Wittebergae: impensis Johannis Helwigii Bibl., Typis Ambrosii Rothii).
Themata medica, De beanorum, archibeanorum, beanulorum & cornutorum quorumque affectibus & curatione, Cornelius Cerastus Cornanus, Cariolinus Tevetius (pseudon.) in *Nugae venales*, 158–78.
Theses de Cochleatione ejusque venenosa contagione, et multiplicibus speciebus, Hasio Leflerus Narragonensis, Volucrinia Lepida Stutzerensis (pseudon.), *in collegii hujus facultatis penetralibus, in frequentia utriusque sexus, Calendis temporis praesentis, praeteriti & futuri* in *Facetiae facetiarum* 1627.
Theses de Hasione et hasibili qualitate, Fabius Stenglec(r)us Leporinus, Lepidus Capito (pseudon.) in *Facetiae facetiarum* 1627; and *Nugae venales*, 93–110.
Vavassor, Franciscus (1722) *De ludicra dictione liber* (Lipsiae). [1658]
Vincent of Beauvois (Vincentius Bellovacensis) (1964 = 1624) *Speculum morale* (Graz: Akademische Druck- und Verlagsanstalt).
Viperano, Giovanni Antonio (1987) *On poetry*, trans. Philip Rollinson (Greenwood: The Attic Press). [1579]
Vulpius (=Volpi), Joannes Antonius (1744) *Liber de Satyrae Latinae natura & ratione, ejusque Scriptoribus qui supersunt, Horatio, Persio, Juvenale* (Patavii: excudebat Josephus Cominus).
Vulteius, Johannes (1619) *Joannes Vulteius Rhemus ad Perosium coecum* in Dornau 1619, 2: 261–2.
Wichgreve, Albert (1627) *Oratio pro Μικανθρωποις sive Homullis* (Francofurti: apud Casparum Rötelium) in *Facetiae facetiarum* 1627.
Wieland, Johann Sebastian (1618a) *Amethystus, continens satyram sobriam adversus cohortem ebriam* (Ulmae: Meder).
Wieland, Johann Sebastian (1618b) *Melissa Satyrica virtute lethargum expellens, ad vigilantiam laboris provocans* [Ulmae: Meder?].

Secondary sources

Abdulla, Adnan K. (1985) *Catharsis in literature* (Bloomington: Indiana University Press).
Anderson, William S. (1982) *Essays on Roman satire* (Princeton: Princeton University Press).
André, J. (1949) *Etude sur les termes de couleur dans la langue Latine* (Paris: Librairie C. Klincksieck).
Baier, Thomas (2005) 'Baldes satirische Dichtungslehre im Zeichen der *Torvitas*', in Freyburger, Gérard and Eckard Lefèvre 2005, 245–55.

Barasch, Moshe (2001) *Blindness: the history of a mental image in Western thought* (New York, London: Routledge).
Barbour, John D. (2004) *The value of solitude: the ethics and spirituality of aloneness in autobiography* (Charlottesville: University of Virginia Press).
Bauer, Barbara (1986) *Jesuitische 'ars rhetorica' im Zeitalter der Glaubenkämpfe*, Mikrokosmos, 18 (Frankfurt am Main: Peter Lang).
Bellandi, Franco (1988) *Persio: Dai 'verba togae' al solipsismo stilistico* (Bologna: Pàtron editore).
Benedek, Thomas G. (1992) 'The influence of Ulrich von Hutten's medical descriptions and metaphorical use of medicine', *Bulletin of the History of Medicine* 66, 3, 355–75.
Bennett, Kenneth C. (1981a) 'The Affective Aspect of Comedy', *Genre* XIV, 2, 191–205.
Bennett, Kenneth C. (1981b) 'The purging of catharsis', *British Journal of Aesthetics* 21, 3, 204–13.
Benzenhöfer, Udo and Wilhelm Kühlmann (1992) *Heilkunde und Krankheitserfahrung in der frühen Neuzeit*, Studien am Grenzrain von Literaturgeschichte und Medizingeschichte, Frühe Neuzeit, 10 (Tübingen: Niemeyer).
Bergdolt, Klaus (1992) *Arzt, Krankheit und Therapie bei Petrarca: die Kritik an Medizin und Naturwissenschaft im italienischen Frühhumanismus* (Weinheim: VCH, Acta humaniora).
Berger, Arnold E. (1931) *Die Sturmtruppen der Reformation. Ausgewählte Flugschriften der Jahre 1520–1525* (Leipzig: Philipp Reclam jun.).
Best, Thomas W. (1969) *The humanist Ulrich von Hutten: a reappraisal of his humour* (Chapel Hill: The University of North Carolina Press).
Best, Thomas W. (1971) 'Introduction', in *Eccius dedolatus*, Thomas W. Best (ed.) (Lexington: The University Press of Kentucky), 13–25.
Billerbeck, Margarethe and Christian Zubler (eds) (2000) *Das Lob der Fliege von Lukian bis L.B. Alberti* (Bern: Peter Lang).
Birney, Alice Lotvin (1973) *Satiric catharsis in Shakespeare: a theory of dramatic structure* (Berkeley: University of California Press).
Blanchard, W. Scott (1995) *Scholars' bedlam: Menippean satire in the Renaissance* (London and Toronto: Bucknell University Press).
Botschuyver, H. J. (1935) *Scholia in Horatium λ φ ψ codicum Parisinorum Latinorum 7972, 7974, 7971* (Amstelodami in aedibus H. A. van Bottenburg N.V.).
Bouchet, Gabriel (1927) *La medicine dans Horace et dans Virgile* (Aubenas: Imprimerie d'éditions médicales).
Bowen, Barbara C. (1998) *Enter Rabelais, laughing* (Nashville: Vanderbilt University Press).
Bramble, J. C. (1974) *Persius and the programmatic satire: a study in form and imagery* (Cambridge: Cambridge University Press).
Braund, S. H. (1988) *Beyond anger: a study of Juvenal's Third Book of Satires* (Cambridge: Cambridge University Press).
Braund, Susanna Morton and Christopher Gill (eds) (1997) *The passions in Roman thought and literature* (Cambridge: Cambridge University Press).
Braund, Susanna Morton (1997) 'A passion consoled? Grief and anger in Juvenal 'Satire' 13', in Braund and Gill 1997, 68–88.
Braund, Susanna Morton and Paula James (1998) '*Quasi homo*: distortion and contortion in Seneca's *Apocolocyntosis*', *Arethusa* 31, 3, 285–311.

Braund, Susanna Morton and Barbara K. Gold (1998) 'Introduction', *Arethusa* 31, 3, 247–56.

Brock, Roger (2000) 'Sickness in the body politic: medical imagery in the Greek polis', in Valerie M. Hope and Eireann Marshall (eds) *Death and disease in the ancient city* (London: Routledge), 24–34.

Brummack, Jürgen (1971) 'Zu Begriff und Theorie der Satire', *Deutsche Vierteljahrsschrift für Literaturwissenschaft und Geistesgeschichte* 45, Mai, 275–377.

Böcking, Eduardus (ed.) (1860) *Ulrichi Hutteni equitis Germani opera quae reperiri potuerunt omnia*, 4 (Lipsiae: in aedibus Teubnerianis).

Carraud, Christophe (2002) 'Commentaires, notes et index' in Petrarch (2002).

Carver, Robert H. F. (2007) *The Protean ass: the Metamorphoses of Apuleius from Antiquity to the Renaissance* (Oxford: Oxford University Press).

Claren, Lutz *et al.* (2003) 'Einleitung', in Jacob Balde SJ, *Urania victrix* (Tübingen: Max Niemeyer Verlag), vii–xli.

Classen, C. J. (1976) 'Barocke Zeitkritik in antikem Gewande. Bemerkungen zu den medizinischen Satiren des "Teutschen Horatius" Jacob Balde S. J.', *Daphnis* 5, 1, 67–125.

Colie, Rosalie L. (1966) *Paradoxia epidemica: the Renaissance tradition of paradox* (Princeton: Princeton University Press).

Colish, Marcia L. (1985) *The Stoic tradition from Antiquity to the early Middle Ages. I. Stoicism in classical Latin literature* (Leiden: E. J. Brill).

Cousins, Norman (ed.) (1982) *The physician in literature* (Philadelphia: The Saunders Press).

De Landtsheer, Jeanine (2000) 'Erycius Puteanus's *Caecitatis consolatio* (1609) and Constantijn Huygens's *Ooghentroost* (1647)', *Humanistica Lovaniensia* 49, 209–29.

De Smet, Ingrid A. R. (1996) *Menippean satire and the republic of letters 1581–1655* (Genève: Librairie Droz).

Desmond, William D. (2006) *The Greek praise of poverty: the origins of ancient cynicism* (Notre Dame, Indiana: University of Notre Dame Press).

Deupmann, Christoph (2002) *'Furor satiricus': Verhandlungen über literarische Aggression im 17. und 18. Jahrhundert* (Tübingen: Niemeyer).

Edwards, Catherine (1999) 'The suffering body: philosophy and pain in Seneca's *Letters*', in James I. Porter (ed.) *Constructions of the classical body* (Ann Arbor: The University of Michigan Press), 252–68.

Engelhardt, Dietrich von (1992) 'Systematische Überlegungen zum Verhältnis von Medizin und Literatur im Zeitalter des Barock', in Benzenhöfer and Kühlmann 1992, 30–54.

Erskine, Andrew (1997) 'Cicero and the expression of grief', in Braund and Gill 1997, 36–47.

Esser, Albert (1961) *Das Anlitz der Blindheit in der Antike: die kulturellen und medizinhistorischen Ausstrahlungen des Blindenproblems in den antiken Quellen* (Leiden: Brill).

Fetkenheuer, Klaus (2001) *Die Rezeption der Persius-Satiren in der lateinischen Literatur. Untersuchungen zu ihrer Wirkungsgeschichte von Lucan bis Boccaccio* (Bern: Lang).

Ficca, Flaviana (2001) *Remedia doloris. La parola come terapia nelle 'Consolazioni' di Seneca* (Napoli: Loffredo editore).

Flemming, Rebecca (2000) *Medicine and the making of Roman women. Gender, nature, and authority from Celsus to Galen* (Oxford: Oxford University Press).

Freudenburg, Kirk (1993) *The walking muse: Horace on the theory of satire* (Princeton: Princeton University Press).

Freudenburg, Kirk (2001) *Satires of Rome: threatening poses from Lucilius to Juvenal* (Cambridge: Cambridge University Press).

Freyburger, Gérard and Eckard Lefèvre (2005) *Balde und die römische Satire / Balde et la satire romaine* (Tübingen: Gunter Narr Verlag).

Frye, Northrop 1973 (1957) *Anatomy of criticism: four essays* (Princeton: Princeton University Press).

Füssel, Marian (2005) 'Riten der Gewalt. Zur Geschichte der akademischen Deposition und des Pennalismus in der frühen Neuzeit', www.burschenschaft.de

Gaisser, Julia Haig (2008) *The fortunes of Apuleius and the Golden Ass: a study in transmission and reception* (Princeton: Princeton University Press).

Garland, Robert (1995) *The eye of the beholder: deformity and disability in the Graeco-Roman world* (London: Duckworth).

Geraldine, M. Sister (1964) 'Erasmus and the tradition of paradox', *Studies in Philology* 61, 41–63.

Gold, Barbara K. (1998) 'The house I live in is not my own': Women's bodies in Juvenal's *Satires*', *Arethusa* 31, 3, 369–86.

Golden, Leon (1973) 'The purgation theory of catharsis', *Journal of Aesthetics and Art Criticism* 31, 4, 473–9.

Gowers, Emily (1993) *The loaded table: representations of food in Roman literature* (Oxford: Clarendon Press).

Hale, David George (1971) *The body politic: a political metaphor in Renaissance English literature* (The Hague, Paris: Mouton).

Hamdorf, F. W. (1964) *Griechische Kultpersonifikationen der vorhellenistischen Zeit* (Mainz).

Hardison, O. B., Jr. (1962) *The enduring moment: a study of the idea of praise in Renaissance literary theory and practice* (Chapel Hill: The University of North Carolina Press).

Hartkamp, Rolf Friedrich (2005) 'Heilkunst oder Hexenküche? Jacob Baldes Zeitkritik in der dritten *Satyra de medicinae gloria*', in Freyburger and Lefèvre 2005, 207–17.

Hathaway, Baxter (1962) *The age of criticism: the late Renaissance in Italy* (Ithaca: Cornell University Press).

Häussler, Reinhard (1978) 'Drei Gedichte an den Schlaf: Statius – Balde – Hölderlin', *Arcadia* 2, 113–45.

Healy, Margaret (2001) *Fictions of disease in early modern England: bodies, plagues and politics* (Basingstoke: Palgrave – now Palgrave Macmillan).

Heitmann, Klaus (1958) *Fortuna und virtus: eine Studie zu Petrarcas Lebensweisheit* (Köln, Graz: Böhlau Verlag).

Hertel, Gerhard (1969) *Die Allegorie von Reichtum und Armut: ein aristophanisches Motiv und seine Abwandlungen in der abendländischen Literatur* (Nürnberg: Verlag Hans Carl).

Hess, Günter (1971) *Deutsch-lateinische Narrenzunft: Studien zum Verhältnis von Volkssprache und Latinität in der satirischen Literatur des 16. Jahrhunderts* (München: C. H. Beck'sche Verlagsbuchhandlung).

Hodges, Devon L. (1985) *Renaissance fictions of anatomy* (Amherst: The University of Massachusetts Press).
Holländer, Eugen (1905) *Die Karikatur und Satire in der Medizin* (Stuttgart: Ferdinand Enke).
IJsewijn, Josef and Dirk Sacré (1998) *Companion to Neo-Latin studies, 2*, Supplementa humanistica Lovaniensia, XIV (Leuven: Leuven University Press).
Jaeger, W. (1957) 'Aristotle's Use of Medicine as Model of Method in his Ethics', *Journal of Hellenic Studies* 77, 54–61.
Jillings, Lewis (1995) 'The Aggression of the Cured Syphilitic: Ulrich von Hutten's Projection of His Disease as Metaphor', *The German Quarterly* 68, 1, 1–18.
Kemper, Hans-Georg (1987) *Deutsche Lyrik der frühen Neuzeit, 2*, Konfessionalismus (Tübingen: Niemeyer).
Kernan, Alvin (1959) *The cankered muse: satire of the English Renaissance* (New Haven: Yale University Press).
Kindermann, Udo (1978) *Satyra. Die Theorie der Satire im Mittellateinischen. Vorstudie zu einer Gattungsgeschichte* (Nürnberg: Verlag Hans Carl).
Kivistö, Sari (2002) *Creating anti-eloquence:* Epistolae obscurorum virorum *and the humanist polemics on style*, Commentationes Humanarum Litterarum, 118 (Helsinki: Societas Scientiarum Fennica).
Kivistö, Sari (2007) 'G. F. von Franckenau's *Satyra sexta* (1674) on male menstruation and female testicles', in Anu Korhonen and Kate Lowe (eds) *The trouble with ribs: women, men and gender in early modern Europe*, COLLeGIUM, Studies across disciplines in the humanities and social sciences 2, 82–102.
Kivistö, Sari (2008a) '*Ars iocandi*: latinankielisiä tutkielmia leikinlaskun taidosta, rajoista ja rangaistavuudesta', in Janna Kantola and Heta Pyrhönen (eds) *Tutkielmia Homeroksesta Hessu Hopoon* (Helsinki: SKS).
Kivistö, Sari (2008b) 'Sour faces, happy lives? On laughter, joy and happiness of the agelasts', in Heli Tissari *et al.* (eds) *Happiness*, COLLeGIUM, Studies across disciplines in the humanities and social sciences 3, 79–100.
Knepper, J. (1904) 'Ein deutscher Jesuit als medizinischer Satiriker. Zum Jubiläum Baldes am 4. Januar 1904', *Archiv für Kulturgeschichte* 2, 38–59.
Könneker, Barbara (1991) *Satire im 16. Jahrhundert: Epoche – Werke – Wirkung* (München: Beck).
Konstan, David (2006) *The emotions of the ancient Greeks: studies in Aristotle and classical literature* (Toronto: University of Toronto Press).
Kühlmann, Wilhelm (1982) *Gelehrtenrepublik und Fürstenstaat: Entwicklung und Kritik des deutschen Späthumanismus in der Literatur des Barockzeitalters* (Tübingen: Max Niemeyer Verlag).
Kühlmann, Wilhelm (1992) 'Selbstverständigung im Leiden: Zur Bewältigung von Krankheitserfahrungen im versgebundenen Schrifttum der Frühen Neuzeit. (P. Lotichius Secundus, Nathan Chytraeus, Andreas Gryphius)', in Benzenhöfer and Kühlmann 1992, 1–29.
Lackenbacher, Hans (1937) 'Persius und die Heilkunde', *Wiener Studien* 55, 1–2, 130–41.
Laín Entralgo, Pedro (1970) *The therapy of the word in classical Antiquity*, L. J. Rather and John M. Sharp (eds, trans) (New Haven: Yale University Press).
Langholf, Volker (1996) 'Lukian und die Medizin: zu einer tragischen Katharsis bei den Abderiten', *ANRW* 37, 3, 2793–841.

Lausberg, Heinrich (1998) *Handbook of literary rhetoric: a foundation for literary study*, Matthew T. Bliss *et al.* (trans) (Leiden: Brill).
Lloyd, G. E. R. (2003) *In the grip of disease: studies in the Greek imagination* (Oxford: Oxford University Press).
Long, A. A. and D. N. Sedley (1987) *The Hellenistic philosophers,* 1. (Cambridge: Cambridge University Press).
Marsh, David (1998) *Lucian and the Latins: humor and humanism in the early Renaissance* (Ann Arbor: University of Michigan Press).
Mayer, Roland (2005) 'Sleeping with the enemy: satire and philosophy', in Kirk Freudenburg (ed.) *The Cambridge companion to Roman satire* (Cambridge: Cambridge University Press), 146–59.
McClure, George W. (1990) *Sorrow and consolation in Italian humanism* (Princeton: Princeton University Press).
Mendell, C. W. (1920) 'Satire as popular philosophy', *Classical Philology* 15, 2, 138–57.
Mertz, James J. *et al.* (eds) (1989) *Jesuit Latin poets of the 17th and 18th centuries: an anthology of neo-Latin poetry* (Wauconda: Bolchazy-Carducci publishers).
Meter, J. H. (1984) *The literary theories of Daniel Heinsius: a study of the development and background of his views on literary theory and criticism during the period from 1602 to 1612,* trans. Ina Swart, Respublica literaria neerlandica, 6 (Assen: Van Gorcum).
Meyer, Guilelmus (1915) *Laudes inopiae, dissertatio inauguralis* (Gottingae: Officina Hubertiana).
Migliorini, Paola (1997) *Scienza e terminologia medica nella letteratura latina di età neroniana. Seneca, Lucano, Persio, Petronio.* Studien zur klassischen Philologie, 104 (Frankfurt am Main: Peter Lang).
Miller, Henry Knight (1956) 'The Paradoxical Encomium with Special Reference to Its Vogue in England, 1600–1800', *Modern Philology* 53, 145–78.
Miller, Paul Allen (1998) 'The bodily grotesque in Roman satire: images of sterility', *Arethusa* 31, 3, 257–83.
Morford, Mark (1973) 'Juvenal's Thirteenth Satire', *The American Journal of Philology,* 94, 1, 26–36.
Mueller, Martin (1966) 'Sixteenth-century Italian criticism and Milton's theory of catharsis', *Studies in English Literature, 1500–1900,* 6, 1, 139–50.
Nauta, G. A. (1931) 'Annotations to W. Map's *De Nugis curialium*', *Neophilologus* 16, 1, 194–6.
Nordenfalk, Carl (1985) 'The five senses in late medieval and Renaissance art', *Journal of the Warburg and Courtauld Institutes* 48, 1–22.
Notter, Catherine (2005) 'Echos de Martial dans la satire des médecins de Jacob Balde', in Freyburger and Lefèvre 2005, 171–88.
Nussbaum, Martha C. (1996) *The therapy of desire: theory and practice in Hellenistic ethics*, 4th edn (Princeton: Princeton University Press).
(*OCD* =) *Oxford classical dictionary,* Simon Hornblower and Antony Spawforth (eds) (New York: Oxford University Press).
Ordine, Nuccio (1996) *Giordano Bruno and the philosophy of the ass* (New Haven: Yale University Press).
Pagrot, Lennart (1961) *Den klassiska verssatirens teori. Debatten kring genren från Horatius t.o.m. 1700-talet* (Stockholm: Almqvist & Wiksell).
Panizza, Letizia A. (1985) 'Active and contemplative in Lorenzo Valla: the fusion of opposites', in Vickers 1985, 181–223.

Pasoli, Elio (1982) *Tre poeti latini espressionisti: Properzio, Persio, Giovenale*, Giancarlo Giardina e Rita Cuccioli Melloni (eds) (Roma: Edizioni dell'Ateneo).

Pease, Arthur Stanley (1926) 'Things without Honor', *Classical Philology* 21, 1, 27–42.

Pernot, Laurent (1993) *La rhétorique de l'éloge dans le monde Gréco-Romain*. Tome II. Les valeurs (Paris: Institut d'Études Augustiniennes).

Perosa, Alessandro (1946) 'Febris: a poetic myth created by Poliziano', *Journal of the Warburg and Courtauld Institutes*, 9 (University of London: The Warburg Institute), 74–95.

Pieters, Jürgen and Lise Gosseye (2008) 'The paradox of paragone: painters and poets in Constantijn Huygens' *Ooghen-Troost*', *Neophilologus* 92, 177–92.

Pisi, Giordana (1983) *Il medico amico in Seneca* (Parma: Università degli studi di Parma, Istituto di lingua e letteratura Latina).

Porter, Roy (ed.) (2001) *Cambridge illustrated history of medicine* (Cambridge: Cambridge University Press).

Porter, Roy and G. S. Rousseau (1998) *Gout: the patrician malady* (New Haven and London: Yale University Press).

Randolph, Mary Claire (1941) 'The medical concept in English Renaissance satiric theory: its possible relationships and implications', *Studies in Philology* 38, 2, 125–57.

Reckford, Kenneth J. (1962) 'Studies in Persius', *Hermes* 90, 476–504.

Reckford, Kenneth J. (1998) 'Reading the sick body: Decomposition and morality in Persius' third satire', *Arethusa* 31, 3, 337–54.

Rée, Jonathan (1999) *I see a voice: a philosophical history of language, deafness and the senses* (London: Harper Collins Publishers).

Relihan, Joel C. (1993) *Ancient Menippean satire* (Baltimore: The Johns Hopkins University Press).

Relihan, Joel C. (1996) 'Menippus in Antiquity and the Renaissance' in R. Bracht Branham and Marie-Odile Goulet-Cazé (eds) *The Cynics: the cynic movement in antiquity and its legacy* (Berkeley: University of California Press), 265–93.

Relihan, Joel C. (2007) *The prisoner's philosophy: life and death in Boethius's Consolation* (Notre Dame, Indiana: University of Notre Dame Press).

Robathan, Dorothy M. and F. Edward Crantz (1976) 'A. Persius Flaccus', in F. Edward Cranz and Paul Oskar Kristeller (eds) *Catalogus translationum et commentariorum*, 3 (Washington: The Catholic University of America Press), 201–312.

Robinson, Christopher (1979) *Lucian and his influence in Europe* (London: Duckworth).

Ronnick, Michele V. (1991) *Cicero's Paradoxa Stoicorum: a commentary, an interpretation and a study of its influence* (Frankfurt am Main: Peter Lang).

Roscher, W. H. (ed.) (1884–1937) *Ausführliches Lexikon der griechischen und römischen Mythologie* (Leipzig: Teubner).

Sallares, Robert (2002) *Malaria and Rome: a history of malaria in ancient Italy* (Oxford: Oxford University Press).

Sanders, Barry (1995) *Sudden glory: laughter as subversive history* (Boston: Beacon Press).

Sanford, Eva M. (1960) 'Juvenalis, Decimus Junius' in Paul Oskar Kristeller (ed.) *Catalogus translationum et commentariorum*, 1 (Washington: The Catholic University of America Press), 175–238.

Sauer, Christoph Friedrich (2005) '*Animosum scribendi genus*. Annäherungen an den Begriff der *Satyra* bei Jacob Balde', in Freyburger and Lefèvre 2005, 13–24.

Sawday, Jonathan (1995) *The body emblazoned: dissection and the human body in Renaissance culture* (London: Routledge).

Scarborough, John (1969) *Roman medicine* (London: Thames and Hudson).

Schäfer, Eckart (1976) *Deutscher Horaz: Conrad Celtis, Georg Fabricius, Paul Melissus, Jakob Balde; die Nachwirkung des Horaz in der neulateinischen Dichtung Deutschlands* (Wiesbaden: Franz Steiner Verlag GmbH.).

Schäfer, Walter Ernst (1992) *Moral und Satire. Konturen oberrheinischer Literatur des 17. Jahrhunderts*, Frühe Neuzeit, 7 (Tübingen: Max Niemeyer Verlag).

Schleusener-Eichholz, Gudrun (1985) *Das Auge im Mittelalter*, 1–2 (München: Wilhelm Fink Verlag).

Schmitz, Heinz-Günter (1972) *Physiologie des Scherzes. Bedeutung und Rechtfertigung der Ars iocandi im 16. Jahrhundert* (Hildesheim: Georg Olms Verlag).

Schnur, Harry C. (ed.) (1967) *Lateinische Gedichte deutscher Humanisten* (Stuttgart: Philipp Reclam jun.).

Scivoletto, Nino (ed.) (1964) *Auli Persi Flacci Saturae* (Firenze: 'La nuova Italia' editrice).

Seidel, Robert (1994) *Späthumanismus in Schlesien: Caspar Dornau (1577–1631), Leben und Werk* (Tübingen: Niemeyer).

Sellars, John (2003) *The art of living: the Stoics on the nature and function of philosophy* (Aldershot: Ashgate).

Sellin, Paul R. (1968) *Daniel Heinsius and Stuart England, with a short-title checklist of the work of Daniel Heinsius* (Leiden: Leiden University Press).

Siraisi, Nancy G. (1990) *Medieval & early Renaissance medicine: an introduction to knowledge and practice* (Chicago, London: The University of Chicago Press).

Siraisi, Nancy G. (2004) 'Oratory and Rhetoric in Renaissance Medicine', *Journal of the History of Ideas*, 65, 2, 191–211.

Spallici, Aldo (1941) *La medicina in Persio* (Milano).

Steiger, Johann Anselm (2005) *Medizinische Theologie: Christus medicus und theologia medicinalis bei Martin Luther und im Luthertum der Barockzeit* (Leiden: Brill).

Stroh, Wilfried (2004) *Baldeana: Untersuchungen zum Lebenswerk von Bayerns grösstem Dichter*, Bianca-Jeanette Schröder (ed.) (München: Herbert Utz Verlag).

Sullivan J. P. (1978) 'Ass's ears and *attises*: Persius and Nero', *American Journal of Philology* 99, 159–70.

Sutton, Dana F. (1994) *The catharsis of comedy* (Lanham and London: Rowman & Littlefield Publishers, Inc.).

Taylor, Samuel S. B. (1988) 'Vis comica and comic vices: catharsis and morality in comedy', *Forum for Modern Language Studies* XXIV, 4, 321–31.

Tieleman, Teun (2003) *Chrysippus' On affections: reconstruction and interpretation*, Philosophia antica, 94 (Leiden: Brill).

Tomarken, Annette H. (1990) *The smile of truth: the French satirical eulogy and its antecedents* (Princeton: Princeton University Press).

Valentin, Jean-Marie (ed.) (1986) *Jakob Balde und seine Zeit: Akten des Ensisheimer Kolloquiums, 15.–16. Oktober 1982* (Bern, Frankfurt am Main, New York: Lang).

Vegetti, Mario (1995) *La medicina in Platone* (Venezia: Cardo).
Vickers, Brian (ed.) (1985) *Arbeit – Musse – Meditation: Betrachtungen zur* Vita activa *und* Vita contemplativa (Zürich: Verlag der Fachvereine).
Vinge, Louise (1975) *The five senses: studies in a literary tradition* (Lund: CWK Gleerup).
Vredeveld, Harry (2001) 'Deaf as Ulysses to the Siren's Song: The Story of a Forgotten Topos', *Renaissance Quarterly* 56, 846–82.
Wagner, Peter (1993) 'The satire on doctors in Hogarth's graphic works' in Marie Mulvey Robert and Roy Porter (eds) *Literature and medicine during the eighteenth century* (London: Routledge), 200–25.
Walters, Jonathan (1998) 'Making a spectacle: deviant men, invective, and pleasure', *Arethusa* 31, 3, 355–67.
Weinberg, Bernard (1961) *A history of literary criticism in the Italian Renaissance*, 1–2 (Chicago: The University of Chicago Press).
Wiegand, Hermann (1992) 'Ad vestras, medici, supplex prosternitur aras: Zu Jakob Baldes Medizinersatiren', in Benzenhöfer and Kühlmann 1992, 247–69.
Wilson, Katharina M. and Elizabeth M. Makowski (1990) *Wykked wyves and the woes of marriage. Misogamous Literature from Juvenal to Chaucer* (Albany: State University of New York Press).
Wilson, Marcus (1997) 'The subjugation of grief in Seneca's "Epistles"', in Braund and Gill 1997, 48–67.
Witke, Charles (1970) *Latin satire: the structure of persuasion* (Leiden: Brill).
Wootton, David (2006) *Bad medicine: doctors doing harm since Hippocrates* (Oxford: Oxford University Press).
Wöhrle, Georg (1991) 'Zur metaphorischen Verwendung von *elkos* und *ulcus* in der antiken Literatur', *Mnemosyne* 44, Fasc. 1–2, 1–16.
Ziolkowski, Jan M. (ed.) (2008) *Solomon and Marcolf* (Harvard: Harvard University Press).

Index

Abderites, 69
Achilles, 76
Aesop, 137, 156, 165
Agesilaus, 76, 146
Agrippinus, 67
Albizzi, Albiera degli, 68
Alcidamas, 129
Alexander the Great, 92, 136, 146, 148
Alphonsus, 80, 125
Anatome joco-seria conscientiae, 2
anatomy, 2–3, 179nn5–6
Anaxagoras, 110, 124
Anaximander, 104
andabatae, 112–13
Anderson, William, 15
Antipater, 111, 115
Antonius, Marcus, 19, 146
Appius Claudius Caecus, 115
Apuleius, 77, 159
Aquinas, Thomas, 154
Archimedes, 125–6
Aristides, 143
Aristophanes, 75, 114, 179n7
Aristotle, 1, 9, 10, 18, 41–3, 48, 49, 51, 91, 103, 110, 120, 145–6, 156, 185n20, 186n26
Asa, King, 76
Asconius Pedianus, Quintus, 115
ass literature, 1, 69, 120–1, 159, 163, 179n2, 191n20, 191n21, 193n6
asthma, 86
Audomarus, 107
Aufidius, Gnaeus, 115
Augustine, 98, 103, 120, 122, 187n9
Augustus, 38, 146
Avenzoar, 63

Bacchus, 77, 78, 134, 135, 136, 139, 166
Badius Ascensius, Jodocus, 21
Balde, Jacob, 8, 11, 172
  Ad somnum, 132
  Agathyrsus, 150–2, 172, 174
  Antagathyrsus, 150, 153–5
  De eclipsi solari, 105, 113
  De studio poetico, 36, 65, 155
  Lyricorum libri, 111, 143
  Medicinae gloria, 12, 17, 35–7, 132
  Satyra contra abusum tabachi, 140
  Silvarum libri, 126, 156
  Solatium podagricorum, 62, 72, 74, 77, 79–80, 82, 84–6, 88–93, 102, 153
  Urania Victrix, 122
  Vultuosae torvitatis encomium, 155–7
Barasch, Moshe, 106
Barclay, John, 110
beards, 143
Bebel, Heinrich, 11
Beer, Johann, 2
Bellerophon, 76
Benedek, Thomas G., 55
Beroaldo, Filippo the Elder, 9, 15, 136, 166
Best, Thomas W., 161
Blanchard, Scott W., 28, 171
blindness, 29–30, 57, 82, 103–19, 122, 127, 158, 171, 190n2
Boethius, Anicius Manlius Severinus, 25, 35, 90, 108–9, 128, 170, 183n4, 190n7
Bonciarius, Marcus Antonius, 117
breath (*pneuma*), 22–3, 57, 72, 86, 133, 134, 135, 137
Britannicus, Johannes, 21, 62, 187n1
Bronzino, Agnolo, 122
bulla, 71–2
Burton, Robert, 3, 179n6

Cajetan, Tommaso de, 70
Calvin, Jean, 155
Candidus, Pantaleon, 78–9
Caracalla, 146, 148
Cardano, Girolamo
  De consolatione, 108

Cardano, Girolamo – *continued*
Medicinae encomium, 63, 65
Podagrae encomium, 28, 80, 91, 93–4
Carnarius, Johannes, 64–5, 74, 77–8, 84, 86, 92, 187n4
Carneades, 110
Casaubon, Isaac, 8, 9, 10, 95
Catadupa, 126
catharsis, 4–5, 16, 37, 38–9, 41–54, 60, 95, 150, 159, 165, 184n12, 184n16
Cato the Elder, 125, 136, 138, 147, 152
Celsus, Cornelius, 20, 24, 25, 39, 99, 189n33
Celtis, Conrad, 10
Cerutus, Federicus, 36–7
Chrysippus of Soli, 5, 10, 67, 110, 137–8, 156
Chytraeus, Nathan, 17, 187n7
Cicero, 1, 4, 5, 7, 65, 118, 141, 154, 170, 191n24, 193n7
De inventione, 113
De natura deorum, 104
De oratore, 83, 144
De re publica, 126
De senectute, 100–1
Tusculanae disputationes, 5–7, 15, 18, 19, 22–3, 84, 88, 97, 98, 107, 108, 109, 111–12, 115, 117, 121, 129, 174, 180n11, 180n12, 182n43, 190n14
Claudius, 68, 141
Cleanthes, 56, 85
cochleatio, 158, 193n5
Codrus Urceus, Antonius, 57, 129
Coiter, Volcher, 121
consolations, 4, 29–30, 73–4, 82, 84, 89, 101–2, 107–8, 119, 131, 139, 190n4
Copernicus, Nicolaus, 156
Cordus, Euricius, 11
Cornelius, 160, 162–3
Crantor, 10
Criep, Willem, 116
Crusius, Martin (Kraus, Martin), 103–4
Cunaeus, Petrus, 37–8, 184n9
Sardi venales, 68–9, 141
Cupid, 113
Cynicism, 10, 156, 182n43
Czanakius, Matthaeus (Czanaki Máté), 94–100

David, 146
deafness, 30, 108, 120–7, 191n23
deformity, *see* dwarfs; ugliness
De Hossche, Sidronius, 132
Demetrius, 115
De Meyere, Lieven, 80–1
Democritus, 1, 10, 69, 109–10, 115
Demodocus, 107, 116
deposition, 59, 161–2
Descartes, René, 118, 121
De Smet, Ingrid, 28
Deupmann, Christoph, 52, 183n1
Dido, 113
Didymus, 116
Diodotus, 116, 190n14
Diogenes, 10, 147, 151, 155
Diomedes, 146
D'Israeli, Isaac, 148
doctors, 11–17, 25, 34–5, 41, 50, 54–5, 58, 60, 63, 91, 111, 172, 180n22, 181n26
Donne, John, 2
Dornau, Caspar, 29
Drant, Thomas, 36
Drexel, Jeremias, 157
dropsy, 22, 133, 134, 182n39
drunkenness, 17, 30, 57, 64, 75, 87, 112, 132–40, 192n38
Dryden, John, 37, 40–1, 44
Du Bellay, Joachim, 122
Duns Scotus, Johannes, 59, 156
dwarfs, 30, 64, 140, 143–9

ears, 19, 56, 85, 111, 120–3, 148, 186n34, 191n20, 191n21
see also deafness
Eccius Dedolatus, 16, 57–60, 161, 166, 171
Ennius, 19, 91, 157
Epictetus, 9, 67
Epicureanism, 46, 47, 77, 83, 84, 98, 109, 140, 152
epideictic rhetoric, *see* eulogies

Epimenides Gnosius, 130
Epistolae obscurorum virorum, 57, 163
Erasmus of Rotterdam, 29, 60, 64, 66, 77, 78, 85, 86, 89, 95, 146, 151, 165, 191n26
eulogies
  disease, 28–30, 63–6
  medicine, 63
  see also individual diseases
eutrapelia, 102
Eve, 104
eyes, 75, 103–11, 114–19, 133–4, 141, 155, 159
  see also blindness

facetiae, 11, 31, 42, 173
facies Hippocratica, 27
Farnaby, Thomas, 9
farts, 142–3, 161, 167–9, 193n7
fatness, *see* obesity
Favorinus, 65, 67
fevers, 5, 6, 13–14, 18, 59, 61, 65, 67–74, 108, 149, 153, 159
Ficino, Marsilio, 146
Fimbria, Gaius, 124, 191n24
Fischart, Johann, 144, 187n5
Fortuna, 113–14
Fracastoro, Hieronymus, 188n10
France, Anatole, 124
Francesi, Matteo, 86
Franck von Franckenau, Georg, 120–1, 129–30
Frischlin, Nicodemus, 4, 10, 16, 55–7, 60, 134–5, 171
Fronto, 129
Frye, Northrop, 3

Galen, 1, 5, 15, 74
Gellius, Aulus, 67, 109
Gnatho, 19
Goclenius, Rudolph, 168
Goethe, Johann Wolfgang von, 8
Gorgias, 4
gout, 18, 28, 62, 70, 72, 74–94, 104, 129, 151, 189n29
Gryphius, Andreas, 189n24
Guther, Jacob (Gouthière, Jacques), 30, 106, 109, 110–15

Harpaste, 112
hatred (*odium*), 23, 43, 48–51, 53, 181n26
Havraeus, Johannes (Havre, Jan van), 105–6, 124, 141–2, 182n35, 190n3
Hegendorff, Christoph, 192n33
  Encomium somni, 130–1
  Laus ebrietatis, 138–9
Heinsius, Daniel, 1, 3, 16, 37
  De satyra Horatiana, 42–53, 184n15, 184n16, 184n17, 186n28
  De tragoediae constitutione, 42, 50
  Laus asini, 1
Hess, Günter, 31
Hessus, Helius Eobanus, 87
Hieron, 92
Hippocrates, 1, 24–5, 63
Hippocratic medicine, 7, 18, 22, 27, 67, 74
Hipponax, 156
Hobbes, Thomas, 119, 144, 191n18
Homer, 88, 107, 116, 129
Horace, 2, 7, 8, 10, 13–14, 19–21, 24–8, 33, 35, 37–41, 44–5, 47, 53, 55, 58, 105, 118, 120, 128, 136, 146, 152, 186n37, 188n22
horns, 143, 161, 164–6
Hutten, Ulrich von, 61, 69–73, 113, 149

ignorance, 7–8, 14, 46, 57, 60, 125, 136
indignation, 37–8, 43, 48–9, 53, 109, 185n20
inebriation, *see* drunkenness
itch, 2, 76, 94–100, 108, 133, 189n33, 189n34
Iustitia, 114

Jerome, 108, 141
Jillings, Lewis, 70, 71
Johnston, Arthur, 101
Jonson, Ben, 44–5, 124
Joubert, Laurent, 67–8, 73, 149–50
Jus potandi, 133, 137
Juvenal, 2, 15, 18, 20, 21, 23, 25–6, 37–41, 44, 46, 48–9, 67, 82, 95, 99, 123, 132–3, 141, 157, 181n28, 182n43, 182n46, 191n23

Kernan, Alvin, 16
kidney stones, 66, 81–2, 86
Konstan, David, 185n20
Kreihing, Johannes, 73–4

Lactantius, 122
Landino, Christoforo, 19, 33, 34, 35, 55, 105, 128, 182n36, 190n2
Lange, Christian, 12, 126, 127, 129
laughter, 42, 46, 48–53
Lauremberg, Johann, 95
Lauremberg, Wilhelm, 143
lethargy, 39, 57, 127–32, 151
Licinius Calvus, Cornelius, 146
Lipsius, Justus, 69, 108
Lombard, Peter of, 156
Lot, 137, 138
Luceius Budius, 156
Lucian, 10, 29, 58, 60, 61, 70, 75, 76, 80, 81
Lucilius, 2, 19, 21–2, 182n36
Lucretius, 35, 111, 157
Luther, Martin, 58, 60, 70, 154–5

Maecenas, 141, 165
Mancinellus, Antonius, 21
Manlius, Titus, 146
Marcolf, 165
Martial, 27, 89–90, 180n22, 189n27
Martianus Capella, 14, 60
McClure, George, 108, 190n5
melancholy, 12, 42, 179n6
Melanchthon, Philip, 103, 123, 146, 155
Melander, Otho and Dionysius, 12
Menander, 113
Menander Rhetor, 66
Menapius Insulanus, Gulielmus, 72–3
Menelaus, 146
Menippus, 10, 69
Messalinus, Catullus, 112
Meter, J. H., 43, 51
Metrodorus, 115
Midas, 120
Minerva, 106
Minturno, Antonio Sebastiano, 3, 32–3, 35, 184n16
mock dissertations, 30–1
Molstetter, Philip, 104, 107, 111, 112, 113, 115
Montanus, Petrus, 181n23
Murmellius, Johannes, 38, 56, 128, 185n18, 186n32

Nashe, Thomas, 2
Nicolasius, Georgius, 134
Noah, 138
noses, 142, 148, 156
Nugae venales, 12, 100, 123, 135, 142, 159, 162–4, 168

obesity, 108, 150–5
Obsopoeus, Vincentius, 133, 135
Oedipus, 76, 106, 107
Ofellus, 44, 45
old age, 100–1, 133
otium, 79, 86, 90, 97–8, 127
Ovid, 28, 89, 157

pain, 6, 13, 23, 28, 33, 41, 54–5, 60, 72, 80–8, 93, 96–8, 129, 156
paleness, 25–7, 60, 106, 133, 137, 149, 166, 183n47, 187n37
Panaetius, 188n22
Pannonius, Janus, 189n23
paradoxes, 28–9, 62–6, 83–4, 90, 107, 109, 135, 170
Paris (prince of Troy), 151
Pasch, Georg, 9, 45, 180n15, 180n19
Passerat, Jean, 115–16
St Paul, 139, 146, 148
Perosa, Alessandro, 68
Perotti, Nicolaus, 185n19
Persius, 15, 19–24, 26–7, 36–8, 40, 44, 54–7, 72, 85, 105, 120–1, 123, 127–8, 132–3, 171, 181n32, 183n47, 185n18, 186n34
Petrarch, 4, 46, 67, 82, 88, 98, 108, 109, 111, 115, 122, 124, 127, 147, 148, 157, 168, 172, 189n29
Petronius, 74, 124
Phaestii, 185n23
Philoctetes, 76, 88
Piccolomini, Enea Silvio, 91
Pirckheimer, Willibald
  Podagrae laus, 61, 76, 79–80, 87–93
plague, 17, 187n7

Plato, 5, 10, 34, 45, 46, 47, 54, 64, 65, 67, 95, 150, 151, 179n10
Plautus, 115
Pliny the Elder, 39, 114, 120
Plutarch, 6, 13, 14, 15–16, 18, 24–5, 26, 34–5, 68, 92–3, 95, 101, 118, 121, 131, 181n27, 192n27
Plutus, 114
podagra, *see* gout
Podagraegraphia, 65, 77–80, 84, 86–9, 91–3, 102, 104, 187n5, 189n26
Poliziano, Angelo, 33–4, 68–9, 189n32
Polymestor, 106
Polyphemus, 25, 106, 112
Pontano, Giovanni Gioviano, 55
Pontanus, Georgius Bartholdus, 76–7
Pontanus, Jacobus, 3, 79, 81–2
Poeticae institutiones, 9, 34–5, 38, 50, 52, 54, 183n3
Posidonius, 84, 138
poverty, 66, 75, 78–80, 83, 94, 114, 147, 150, 155
praises, *see* eulogies
Prüschenk von Lindenhofen, Christian Friedrich, 162
Puteanus, Erycius, 116–19, 191n17
Pythagoreanism, 42–5, 79, 156, 159

quartan fever, *see* fevers
Quintilian, 45, 65, 118

Rabus, Jacob, 16, 55–7
Randolph, Mary Claire, 32, 54–5
Rappolt, Friedrich, 7, 45, 49
Ravisius Textor, Johannes, 116, 122, 191n5
Raynaud, Théophile, 148
Relihan, Joel C., 11, 108, 128
Rigault, Nicolas, 21–2, 26, 38–9, 53, 69, 182n46, 183n49
Robortello, Francesco, 10, 41–2, 49–50, 51, 184n16, 185n23

Sanders, Barry, 144
Sardanapalus, 98
scabies, *see* itch
Scaliger, Julius Caesar, 39–40
Schoock, Marten, 120–7, 157, 193n7
Schrevel, Ewald, 1
Semonides, 125
Seneca the Younger, 4, 9, 170, 181n26
Apocolocyntosis, 68, 141, 174
De beneficiis, 13
De consolatione ad Marciam, 24, 83, 117, 181n28
De constantia sapientis, 13–14
De otio, 90
De remediis fortuitorum, 107–8
De tranquillitate animi, 95
De vita beata, 83, 153
Epistulae morales, 6–7, 17, 20, 22–4, 27, 74, 82–4, 86, 89–90, 97, 101, 105, 112, 117, 123–4, 126–7, 138, 141, 147, 151–3, 157, 165, 173–4, 180n13
Quaestiones naturales, 118
Sennert, Daniel, 15, 39, 41, 97, 118, 129, 130, 168, 170, 189n35
seven sleepers of Ephesus, 130, 192n32
skin, 3, 21–3, 25, 54, 56, 59, 87, 95, 152
sleep, *see* lethargy
Socrates, 10, 29, 37, 44, 45, 46–7, 84, 95, 156, 185n18
Stesichorus, 106, 115, 116
Stoicism, 4, 5, 7, 10, 15, 18–19, 29, 42, 44, 46–7, 52, 82–5, 90, 96, 109, 110, 113, 121, 131, 136, 137, 140, 151, 152–4, 156, 167, 174, 183n7
see also Chrysippus, Cicero, Seneca
Straton, 92
students, 20, 24, 31, 97, 128, 158–66
Suetonius, 118
Synesius, 143

Tacitus, 117, 146
Thamyras, 106, 115, 116
therapy, 7, 30, 34, 39, 54–60, 84–5, 161, 165–6, 171
Thersites, 156, 165
thinness, 71, 149–55
Thucydides, 17
thumbs, 126
Tiberius, 124, 137
Timoleon of Corinth, 115

Tiresias, 106–7, 115, 116
Todi, Jacopone da, 103, 122
Tomarken, Annette H., 28, 72, 131–2, 142, 187n7, 188n20

ugliness, 30, 50–1, 144, 155–7
see also dwarfs
Ulysses, 76, 123, 127, 146, 191n23

Vadian, Joachim, 10
Varro, 10, 113
Vavassor, Franciscus, 37
venereal diseases, 66, 93, 95, 187n8, 189n33
Viperano, Giovanni Antonio, 53–4, 186n30
Virgil, 24, 152, 157
Volpi, Giovanni Antonio, 16, 40, 45–9, 53
Vulteius, Johannes, 115

Wichgreve, Albert, 140, 143–9, 168
Wieland, Christoph Martin, 179n2
Wieland, Johann Sebastian, 128, 132–3
Wilson, Marcus, 7, 13
Wireker, Nigellus, 159, 163
wounds, 18, 23–5, 27, 34, 54, 59, 69, 96, 99, 105, 135–6, 151, 158, 182n42–5

Xanthippus, 148
Xenarchus, 116
Xenophon, 189n34

Zeno, 138